BURNING BRIGHT

Rituals, Reiki & Self-Care to Heal
Burnout, Anxiety & Stress

KELSEY J. PATEL

HARMONY BOOKS / NEW YORK

TO MY MOM

whose very own pain and suffering gave
me the gift of healing my own.

AND TO AP

whose patience and grounding love
have been the greatest gifts
of my life.

All rights reserved.
Published in the United States by Harmony Books, an imprint of
Random House, a division of Penguin Random House LLC, New York.
harmonybooks.com

Harmony Books is a registered trademark, and the Circle colophon is
a trademark of Penguin Random House LLC.

Library of Congress Cataloging-in-Publication Data
Names: Patel, Kelsey, author.
Title: Burning bright : rituals, Reiki, and self-care to heal burnout,
anxiety, and stress / Kelsey Patel.
Description: New York : Harmony Books, 2020.
Identifiers: LCCN 2019042067 (print) | LCCN 2019042068 (ebook) |
ISBN 9780593136805 (board) | ISBN 9780593136812 (epub).
Subjects: LCSH: Burn out (Psychology) | Anxiety—Treatment. |
Reiki (Healing system). Classification: LCC BF481 .P374 2020 (print) |
LCC BF481 (ebook) | DDC 158.7/23—dc23.
LC record available at https://lccn.loc.gov/2019042067
LC ebook record available at https://lccn.loc.gov/2019042068

ISBN 9780-593-13680-5
Ebook ISBN 978-0-593-13681-2
Proprietary ISBN 978-0-525-61741-9

Printed in the United States of America

Illustrations by Woolypear

10 9 8 7 6 5 4 3 2 1

CONTENTS

AN INVITATION iv

AN INVITATION

I don't always make the best choices, but today I choose compassion over intolerance, sympathy over hatred, and love over fear.

—L. J. VANIER, CANADIAN PHILOSOPHER AND THEOLOGIAN

My journey began with back pain—searing, debilitating back pain. The more I ignored it, the worse it got. The more I pushed through it, the more paralyzed I felt. I was in my early twenties, and I didn't connect this pain to my crushing stress, my high-pressure job, my troubled family, my toxic boyfriend, my pushing, my exhaustion, or my unwillingness or inability to express any of my deep feelings. I just thought, "My back hurts. Gotta push through."

I was so wrong.

YOU HAVE A CHOICE

What I now know is, there is a path out of pain, anxiety, burnout, fear, grief, sadness, and that feeling of complete overwhelm. When I was experiencing the peak of my back pain, I had no idea that repressed emotions and the stress they cause could manifest as physical pain. I had no idea that my pain could have had anything to do with my exhaustion and burnout, my desperate need for change, my endless list of to-dos, and my feeling that nothing in my life would ever change. I remember complaining about my back to my father, a physical therapist, and he said, "Maybe it's stress." I'd never heard of stress causing pain. I thought everybody had stress, but obviously not everybody had back pain so severe they sometimes questioned whether they could go on living.

Back then, I didn't get it. Now I know that what finally cured my back pain wasn't a drug or physical exercise or surgery or any other external intervention. What cured my back pain was acknowledging the truth of how I was living, becoming aware of how out of harmony my life was, and finally giving myself permission to recognize that my life was my choice and that I also had the choice to do something different. This led me to seek out the energy healing practices that helped get my body, my health, my mind, and my emotions back into alignment—Reiki, EFT, yoga, and other practices you will read about in this book.

I'll tell you more about my path throughout this book, but suffice it to say that I wasted a lot of time looking outside of myself for answers to my problems and cures for my pain. It was only when I looked inside that I saw what was happening in my life and owned it. That's when I understood what was wrong for the first time: I was trying to control everything about my existence so it would be "okay." I was refusing to admit any of my uncomfortable feelings. I was denying my true nature. I was living as the person I thought I was supposed to be, rather than the person I really was. What I needed to do, I finally realized, was to let go, to surrender, to admit, to acknowledge, to accept, and to be myself—my true self, no matter what anyone else expected. To move at my own pace, live in my own way, and nurture the inner flame that had almost been extinguished deep inside me.

That was the beginning, not just of my healing, but of my freedom. That was how I learned that I could shine my own light from my own heart without shame or hesitation. It didn't happen overnight. It happened slowly, over the course of years, as I learned and grew and shifted, bit by bit, trying new practices, working with new teachers, and always questioning: Is this me? Is this right? Is this what I believe? Is this where I want to go? As I kept moving away from external pressures and toward myself, my body changed. As I took more pressure off myself to do and achieve and prove my worth to everyone but myself, my pain faded. As I practiced saying no to the things that didn't serve my greater good, my mind (and my schedule) cleared. As I stopped expecting perfection from myself, I gained confidence, compassion, patience for my journey, and kindness. As I made myself and my health my number one priority, my daily joy increased exponentially. And when I finally recognized myself in the mirror again, I realized that I could turn around and help others find their way back to themselves, too.

Right now, you might feel stressed, overwhelmed, anxious, fearful, sad, in physical pain, or just completely burned out. There is help for you here. This book is not a magical cure for burnout and it's not going to suddenly erase all your pain or anxiety, but what it will do is help you look within to find your own magical cure. Your impulse may be to deny your pain, avoid it, fight it, numb it, freeze it, medicate it, or believe you have no choice but to endure it. When you give yourself permission to use tools to start shifting your energy, you can meet yourself in the actual physical present moment and honor where you are right now.

Your mind will always have you believing that you just have to do a few more things, or maybe even just one more thing, to finally be happy, at peace, healthy, successful, worthy, and joyful. Do you feel that you are so close to happiness, but you can't maneuver those last few steps? You don't need to step outside yourself to reach happiness. You need to follow the path that leads you inside yourself. We are going to work on you finding your peace and your joy and your burning bright, even when stress is part of your life. You're never going to completely eliminate stress because sometimes stress comes from the outside, but you have infinite resources within you that can help you manage it so it doesn't cause harm. Without anything else in your life changing, you can find harmony in your body, mind, and spirit. You don't have to get anywhere or achieve anything first. You are already there. Just as you are right now, you can start burning bright.

But in order to start negotiating with your stress, I want you to understand how powerful and relentless stress can feel and why you experience it the way you do, even if your stress response is different from anyone else's. I want you to see the pain stress causes, not just in you but in your family, your friends, your community, your country, and the world. We're going to bring awareness to stress and what it does in your body—how it launches you into fight, flight, or freeze mode, which can make you angry, or in denial, or paralyzed and unable to move forward in life.

Stress can put you on constant alert, so you become ready to pounce on (fight) anyone who makes a "wrong" comment. Stress can cause you to avoid any confrontation (flight) because you are so afraid of speaking your truth that you run away from who you really are and how you really feel. Stress can keep you stuck in a job or a relationship or a place you loathe (freeze).

Stress can kill dreams and aspirations, or make them feel so unattainable that you stop chasing them. It can make you resentful. It can make you so concerned about everything outside of yourself (like the environment or politics or whatever it is you use as an excuse not to look inward) that you can't see that sometimes what happens outside you mirrors what is happening within. It can take you out of your body, out of the present moment, and separate you from your own core being, your own wise inner voice, your own intuition.

You don't have to experience any of that. You have a choice. In this safe place, we're going to look underneath all those heavy feelings you have, even if you haven't been allowing yourself to feel them. We're going to do a deep dive into *you*, to see what emotions, memories, and patterns are going on that have spiraled into those painful impulses you experience from stress. We're going to figure out what it all means for your life. We're going to think about what your pain tells you about who you are trying to be, and what it says about who you really are . . . and aren't. We're going to figure out what you would rather be feeling and doing and being than what you are feeling and doing and being right now. And then you can make a choice: Do you want to be who you think you should be or do you want to be who you really are? Do you want to live in fear or do you want to live in love?

You deserve a life of harmony and health. You deserve a life of fulfillment and fullness. And you can have it. All those things you want, those things you dream about, those things that are hard for you to even admit you dream about, are accessible to you. We're going to get you connected to how you want to feel. Your direction will become clear. No more fighting. No more fleeing. No more freezing.

We may live in an age of anxiety, but in this book we'll create a space for us to work together. You can choose to live in a wondrous age of physical, mental, and spiritual freedom, in which you live your own life and not anyone else's life, with ease and grace and personal responsibility for everything you feel and do and desire. If you've had anxiety or burnout for a while, this will be a process. I still struggle with anxiety myself—I regularly sense anxiety or overwhelm creeping into my mind, but it's easier now for me to move through it because I have learned to take responsibility for my needs. I have tools to work with my fear, instead of letting it override my whole system and take control of my mind.

In this book, I'll share those same strategies and tools with you, and as you align with your priorities, you'll watch your joyful life unfold. All the noise and chaos trying to get your attention will fade away. You will learn, step by step, just as my students and clients have—just as I have—to be you, and nobody else. And it will be delicious.

So welcome, beautiful one. I invite you into the sacred space generated by this book, where we will build a solid ground on which you can feel safe, ready, and supported, and from which you'll feel sturdy enough to explore the true nature of your limitless self. In this expansive space, I want to help you give yourself permission to feel your feelings, to trust yourself to do less, and to believe in your own intuition. You will heal and grow into the existence that is most in harmony with who you really are, what you came here for, and what you want your life to be. Exploring the micro-changes I suggest in this book with curiosity, and trying out these spiritual practices, can create a macro-shift in your daily life.

~~~~~~

WHAT ARE YOU MADE FOR?

Does it sound too good to be true, that you already have everything you need—that you don't need to expend any effort looking outside yourself for answers because you really can "effort" less to get more out of your life? I was once skeptical, too. It's funny, but all the tools, practices, and techniques I now hold so dear and teach to so many others are things I once found ridiculous.

I grew up in the red state of North Dakota in a very Catholic family. We didn't talk much about feelings. I was brought up to believe that the doctor had more answers about my pain than I did and that if a doctor didn't know about it, it wasn't worth my time. There was the body and its health. There was the mind and its stability. And there was the spirit, which was what you worked on when you went to church every Sunday. None of them had anything to do with the others.

Until I was an adult, I didn't know anything about Reiki or other forms of energy healing. I didn't waste my time with spiritual yoga, and I thought meditation was something people in other countries did. I didn't write feelings in a journal, I didn't spend any time in self-contemplation, and beyond the church services I loved, I certainly didn't ritualize anything in my life. Many of the practices you will learn about in this book were just as foreign to me when I started them.

When I first heard about some of these things, I (like many of my students today) was a true skeptic. When my friends started to tell me they were meditating, I almost scoffed at it. When I heard about energy healing, I thought it was BS. Yoga? Meh. Only if it's a good workout. This is a normal reaction to something new and unfamiliar. What I didn't realize was that these practices were paths to self-awareness and healing beyond my wildest dreams.

Since those early days, I've learned a lot and found many answers. I've been able to help guide thousands of other people through their own transformations, shifts, and healing in ways they never would have believed possible, by using the ancient tools and practices and knowledge I share with you in this book. My own life experience with pain, burnout, anxiety, overwhelm, and pushing myself to the breaking point led me down a path that is finally in line with who I really am and who I want to be. I'm not made for the high-pressure corporate world. I'm made to be a teacher, guide, spiritual empowerment coach, motivational speaker, and energy healer. Without these practices, I never would have discovered that truth about myself.

What are *you* made for?

I have been where you are, and I have come out on the other side stronger and freer than I ever was before. I had to help myself first, and that is what I want to help you do, too. It has become my mission and purpose in life to guide other people to come into their own light by inspiring them to relate to and connect with who they really are, beneath all the noise and clamor of life in a high-pressure world.

I want you to feel able to live your life with purpose, joy, and balance, free of all the things that separate you from your true, precious, beautiful, benevolent self. No matter how anxious, scared, sad, frustrated, or burned out you feel right now, we're going to get you burning bright. To me, burning bright is the opposite of burning out. Burnout comes from excessive, relentless doing, but the beauty of burning bright is that it is not about doing anything more at all. It's really the opposite. It's about learning how to know and trust deep within that all you desire is already inside you, and once you give yourself permission to unlock your heart and get free from the prison of your mind, you will understand that there's nothing more for you to "do." You can simply be, and that is your everything.

When you have burnout, it always feels like there is more to do and more, more, more that you must give. In this book, I want you to see and feel that you are enough without any more doing. Instead, burning bright is about outwardly doing less, and, when you let go, how much more can come into your life—such as unlimited love that, once you access it, will help you to breathe a huge sigh of relief because you will realize that you have always been enough. That there is nothing else to do but be who you are.

When you are burning bright, you will feel a renewed surge of energy, clarity, and light. You will feel able to do everything you want to do with a sense of joyful, easy, and graceful commitment to your path. You will wake up in the morning ready and eager to start the day, without needing to control what comes. You'll embrace your work, your loved ones, and your life. You'll feel a sense of trust in yourself and your path and life's bounty and support for you. You can be the bright flame at the center of a life of peace, love, health, and abundance.

To burn bright is the opposite of the manic, overwhelmed,

anxious, stress-driven, worried energy so many of us associate with productivity and achievement. It is a clean, calm, pure energy, based in love rather than fear—an energy that you can relax into, that feels timeless and dependable and as if it will never run out. It is an endless fountain of contentment that enhances and colors your participation in your own life.

The word you associate with burning bright will be your own. How do you feel when you wake up in the morning, throughout the day, and at night? Right now, think of the word that describes or represents how you would *like to* feel in your life every day, even if it feels incredibly far away right now. You can even close your eyes for a moment and tune in. What word or feeling did you get? That's your burning bright.

For me, when I was in the midst of true burnout, I never felt free. I felt stuck with my back pain, with my family turmoil, with my stressful career, with my toxic on-again, off-again boyfriend. So, burning bright to me has always been about feeling free—to remember that I always have a choice, that I am powerful, and that I can always make changes that support me and my life. That I am never stuck with what life has given me.

We're going to clear a path for you to connect to the radiant health and well-being you deserve, your innate passions and purpose, and your deepest truth, so you can figure out why you are here, and then get out there and live according to that purpose. Throughout this process, I'm going to ask you to keep looking inward, to find new layers of trust and recognition within yourself.

As you hold this book in your hands, know that I have infused it with healing and balancing Reiki energy just for you. The experience of reading this book in any form is intended to open you up to love and permission to burn bright. There is a magic and a divinity to this book—on paper, this book has things to share with you and I wrote these words for you. But what you won't see is the healing and light that this book carries within it, to be with you on your journey. When you hold this book in your hands, have it in your bag, on your desk, or next to your bed—even if you are reading it from an electronic device or listening to it in your car—know that I am connecting with you directly and on purpose. I am sending you blessings and healing from where I am to where you are. I am sending you access to your own courage and to your inner knowledge that you are deeply worthy of all you desire. This book is tangible and intangible. Even the team who helped write and edit this book shared with me that they could feel their energy shifting as they worked with it. You don't need to know where this book is going to take you. Just know that it will take you where you need to go.

Whatever it took to get you here, whatever you did to become willing to do this work for yourself, congratulations. That is huge. I am elated that you have chosen to spend this time with me, and honored to share this experience with you. I have so much yumminess for you here—the ideas, the energy, the grace, the magic, and all that exists between and beyond the words on these pages.

If you accept the invitation and decide that we can work together to go deep inside and release what hurts you, controls you, and limits you, then there is nothing you can't do. The luminous gift of this work is the recognition that you already have everything you need to free yourself. You are in the right place, at the right time, for the right reason. All the things that brought you here had to happen so you could arrive in this moment. No matter how you feel right now, know that you haven't done anything wrong. Your imbalances, disharmonies, fears, and pain come only from not seeing yourself in all your fullness, completeness, rightness, and imperfect perfectness.

This book has three parts. In the first part, we'll explore the mess of being human, with all it entails: the stress, anxiety, and pain of life in the modern world, along with the many ways our experiences imprint on us and make us who we are in seemingly indelible ways. And yet, you can rekindle the flame deep within you, that you knew as a child was part of who you are. You are still that person. You still possess that flame. You can reclaim your joy and your energy with new tools and with deep growth.

In part 2, we'll work on all the ways to excavate your joy. I'll introduce you to techniques and methods of rethinking your body, your mind, and your spirit, for a fuller and brighter experience of life, love, work, and connection. You'll learn about many of the practices I use daily on myself and that I teach to thousands of others, including emotional freedom technique, or EFT (also known as "tapping"), to release pent-up negative energy, and Reiki, the most powerful energy-healing technique I know.

Reiki is based on ancient practices but was first systematized in the nineteenth century in Japan by Dr. Mikao Usui, after a spiritual awakening he experienced while meditating, fasting, and praying on Mount Kurama. He went on to develop the healing practice of Usui Reiki, and opened a Reiki clinic in Tokyo in 1922. He passed on the knowledge to several masters he trained, and the techniques of Reiki have been passed on through a lineage of masters and evolved into a powerful and relevant practice anyone can utilize right now in the twenty-first century.

Reiki utilizes the flow of life energy that exists everywhere all around us and within all beings. We all have Reiki energy within us, and each one of us will experience it in a different way, but anyone can learn how to channel it to ease pain, calm anxiety, and bring positive energy and light into any being, any room, and any situation. I'll show you how you can benefit from these and many other practices to help yourself out of the darker places and into the light whenever you need them.

Finally, in the third part of the book, I'll share my favorite rituals celebrating daily life, big events, and the cyclical nature of earthly existence. From the dramatic to the subtle, these rituals will help you make your life feel more sacred. I'll also share some additional practices with you, from working with crystals to yoga to my personal take on astrology, so you have tools to manage any situation that might come your way. Speaking of my personal take, it's important that you know that the practices and information you will find in this book are rooted in both my personal life experiences with burnout, anxiety, and chronic pain, and the work I've done with thousands of clients and students. This is what I have seen and experienced in more than a decade of helping others to address and relieve these conditions. I know what pain and struggle feel like in this life. I am right here with you.

And finally, what I want you to know before we begin, most deeply and from the depths of your soul, is that you are made for greatness. Everything that you seek is already inside of you and my deepest desire is for you to see how incredibly worthy you are right now of living a life you love and knowing what it truly feels like to be happy, healthy, and abundant.

I know how hard this is. Two days before I signed and got my book deal, I completely self-sabotaged. I didn't believe I was worthy of receiving a book deal and I had to sit in my own fear and physical pain prior to that all-important meeting with the publisher who would ultimately love and accept this book. Even though I didn't feel worthy, I was. And so are you. We all are here to burn bright, and it is our birthright. If you take nothing else away from this book, please take this.

I also want you to know that the secret to burning bright is to accept that *change and shifting and letting go are your new best friends*. These are the keys to freedom, so get ready! We're going to shake things up and knock things loose and move you out of your ruts and into a life that brings you joy.

To prepare your mind and heart for this work, I have created a self-discovery agreement that I would like you to read out loud, commit to in your heart, and sign. First, let's take a moment to prepare. This is something I do in many of my workshops and classes to help create a mutual intention and quiet space from which to start our journey together. We're going to agree on some things, so let's get our minds and hearts aligned.

Find a quiet place where you can sit or lie down comfortably. Lower the lights. Light a candle or some incense. Get comfortable.

Take three slow, deep breaths, inhaling for three counts, and exhaling for three to five counts. In your mind or out loud, say these words:

I give myself permission to engage in self-discovery.

I give myself permission to receive the energy healing this book offers me.

I give myself permission to acknowledge and recognize my worth and my innate value in this world and my worthiness to live a life of radiant health, abundance, and love.

Bring your palms together in front of your heart in a prayer position, and take just a few minutes to sit and breathe and bask in a feeling of gratitude for the good things and blessings you have today, including the ability to explore your own consciousness as you seek out a life more in line with who you really are.

NOW YOU ARE READY.

Please read the following agreement out loud, allowing it to land in your heart space. When the moment feels right and you agree in your heart to the items on this list, sign it, date it, and consider it your sacred vow and deliberate intention for the experience to come. This is the beginning of a spectacular journey into the infinite depths of *you*.

SELF-DISCOVERY
AGREEMENT

~~~

✦ I, _____, do hereby declare my
willingness to participate in the experience of healing.

✦ I understand that I am worthy of the shifts, awareness,
and upliftment available to me through the practices
within this book, and I choose to embody compassion
for myself as I begin this journey.

✦ I permit myself to see myself in all my light, without
judgment, comparison, or the pressure to change any
part of myself.

✦ I give myself permission to receive what I need from
this book and to burn bright.

✦ I choose to give myself the time, space, and love I
require to discover my deepest truths.

✦ I vow to allow change into my life where I most need it
and desire it.

✦ I agree that I can fully acknowledge and accept my
deepest desires.

✦ I promise myself that I am worthy of taking up space in
this world and living a life I love.

✦ I swear to myself that I deserve to be the best version of myself without apology for the bigness of my energy, potential, and beauty.

✦ I grant myself full and unlimited permission to go through this book with love, compassion, and patience with myself.

✦ I admit that I possess profound inner wisdom that can lead me to the answers I seek.

✦ I accept that this book is a resource and an aid, filled with energy and light coming through it to allow me to see myself better.

✦ I acknowledge that what I need to burn bright is already within me.

✦ I acknowledge that all the things I seek are also seeking me.

✦ To these vows, I now commit my energy and will, with infinite compassion for myself, and for my highest good and the good of all beings.

SIGNATURE: _____

DATE: _____

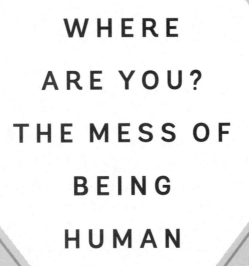

PART

1

WHERE
ARE YOU?
THE MESS OF
BEING
HUMAN

CHAPTER ONE

Awareness:
The Age of Anxiety

We don't see things as they are;
we see them as we are.

ANONYMOUS

THE EARTHQUAKE HIT when I was sitting in my twenty-second-floor apartment in Los Angeles, all alone in my bedroom. My husband was away in another country and, suddenly, the whole building started rocking back and forth. I was literally swaying in the sky, twenty-two floors off the ground, in the middle of the city. I panicked. My palms started sweating, my heart started racing, and all the terrible thoughts started running through my head: Is this the Big One? Is it all over? Is California going to break off into the sea? Am I going to die? *Are we all going to die?*

This was a moment of stress, and I've had plenty of them in my life. Fortunately, I was prepared. On the inside, some deep intuitive part of me knew that my physical body was having a fear response, and there was only one thing I could do: Feel it. I heard a voice in my head saying, "You're safe. It's okay to feel this." I didn't want to feel this fear, but the only other option was to deny it, and to deny a feeling is to repress it, so it stays inside you and doesn't leave.

Of course I was afraid—I was in a situation I couldn't control. I can't control an earthquake. I can't control a swaying building. I can't control what happens to California, or even to myself, in a situation like this. Even through my fear, I knew that whatever was going to happen was going to happen, and there was nothing I could do about it. But there was one thing I could control: my response.

So I chose to ride out the feeling, rather than hanging on to it. I gave myself permission to feel my fear. I let it wash over me and pass through me. I brought my full awareness to what was happening to me at that moment. I stayed present. I kept thinking, "I'm experiencing an earthquake." That was the truth.

And then it was over. It turned out *not* to be the Big One. My building did not come crashing down. California did not break off and sink into the ocean. I was just fine.

As soon as the tremors stopped, I reached out for connection. I checked in with my best friends, who also live in Los Angeles. I told them I was scared. I let them love and support and coddle me a little, because that's what friends are for. One of my girlfriends suggested that we go for a hike, so we met up and I reconnected with the earth, with nature, and with people who bring me a sense of calm. My fear faded. It had been like the wave of an ocean—rising up, peaking, then falling away.

But what if my building had collapsed? It's taken me a long time to get to the place where I can finally say, *That would have been fine, too*. If that's what was going to happen, there would be no point in fighting it. If it's my time, it's my time. I'm happy that it wasn't my time, that I lived to see another day. But if it had been my time, I wouldn't have been able to control that, so what good does it do to try? The lesson, which I have learned again and again in my life, is that the only thing you can control is your own response to fear. When your response is to experience it with full awareness, flowing with it instead of fighting it, that is the remedy.

But where does fear come from?

~~~~

THE SOURCE OF FEAR

Here's a riddle for you, my friend: What do 75 percent of adults say they have had in the past month? Here are some clues: Women have it more than men, it leads to sleepless nights and health problems like chronic pain and upset stomach, it kills sex drive, it makes people overeat, and it can cause anxiety, depression, irritability, anger, constant worrying, and panic attacks. Scary, right?

But there's more. Eighty percent of people have it at work, and 40 percent have it to the extreme. It costs employers $300 billion every year, it lowers job performance, and younger generations are experiencing it more than they ever have before. It's a serious health concern for teenagers in ninth to twelfth grade, and millennials seem to have it the worst. Financial problems often trigger it (even in millionaires), followed by work problems and family responsibilities, and the way most people deal with it is to self-medicate with caffeine, nicotine, prescription medications, alcohol, or long hours in front of a television or online.[1] Even considering all that, it's not always a bad thing, but too much for too long can seriously harm you, if you don't know what to do about it.

Did you guess what it is? It's stress, of course. If you experience chronic stress, my dear, it is standing in your way, generating fear, triggering anxiety, burning you out, pulling you down, damaging your health, clouding your mind, keeping you in a state of grief, and interfering with your connection to your deep inner self, the people in your life, and even your energetic connection to a higher power. Many people don't realize how badly they have it. When I was the most stressed in my life, I probably would have told you I didn't have any stress at all. But I have been stress's unknowing victim and my suffering was extreme. Maybe yours feels extreme to you, too.

But we're going to take on stress because we all deserve a better life than the one we get when we live with stress as our constant, relentless companion. Stress is like the worst roommate you ever had. It constantly harasses you, gnaws at you, keeps you from thinking straight. It brings up all kinds of ridiculous things to worry about. It criticizes you and steals your confidence and makes you feel as if you need it to be successful just to survive.

I have been working on stress with thousands of clients and students for over a decade. The absolute majority of them tell me, when we first begin working together, that they experience some sort of stress, and they are seeking relief from it. And this is what I want to work on with you. Let's knock stress down to size, so you can stop being controlled by it and move on to the bigger and better work of burning bright in your life.

~~~~~

WHAT STRESS REALLY IS AND WHAT IT REALLY DOES

If you have stress, or any of its complications, like chronic pain, an autoimmune disease like Hashimoto's, a chronic condition like fibromyalgia, a hormonal imbalance, an anxiety disorder or clinical depression, confusion about your life purpose, problems in your relationships, a feeling of burnout in your work or personal life, or a constant feeling of overwhelm, you may be stuck in a chronic stress cycle. If you believe that you have to keep pushing and trying and doing and striving and effort-ing, or else you'll fail or lose your grip on everything you've worked for, or disappoint someone, then we have some work to do. Let's get into stress, so we can dismantle it from the inside out.

According to the Oxford dictionary, stress is a state of mental or emotional strain or tension resulting from adverse or demanding circumstances. In other words, stress is a physical response to a momentary experience. Sounds simple enough, right? Something bad or scary or new happens, and it makes you tense because, somehow or other, you're going to have to respond to that situation.

This is actually a good thing, because the physical reaction you experience from stress helps you deal with the problem. This happens with the help of your autonomic nervous system—that's the part of your nervous system that acts without you telling it what to do. It's automatic, and it has two parts: the sympathetic nervous system and the parasympathetic nervous system.

When something threatens you, your sympathetic nervous system is the first responder, turning on the "fight, flight, or freeze" response. When this happens, your neurons send the signal to your adrenal glands to release hormones like adrenaline and cortisol that activate your body so you can respond more quickly and instinctually to danger: Your pupils dilate, you sweat, and your heart rate and blood pressure go up so you have more oxygen and nutrients available for your brain and muscles. Your liver releases glucose for quick energy, your lungs dilate so you can get more oxygen into your blood, and your blood is diverted from your organs and into your muscles so you can move faster and more powerfully.

You also basically stop digesting, fighting off germs, being able to pee, being fertile, and even thinking logically. This is why you can suddenly react more quickly, jumping out of the way of that speeding bus almost before you know you saw it, or lifting the car off the child before thinking logically that you could never do that, or running away from the charging rhino without calculating the relative speed of a human versus a rhino . . . or whatever other drastic thing you have to do to save yourself or somebody else. Without the stress response, humans probably never would have survived the Stone Age, so thank goodness we have it!

But there are two parts to the stress response, and they are supposed to balance each other. The parasympathetic nervous system turns off all those extreme responses in your body—because you can't live in that running-from-a-rhino state all the time. When your brain recognizes that the stressful event is over, it flips the switch to the "rest, digest, and restore" response. This triggers the release of calming hormones, like prolactin, oxytocin, and acetylcholine. The stress hormones get processed out of your system and your pupils, heart rate, blood pressure, and lungs all go back to their normal state again. You get a nice feeling of relaxation, calm, and euphoria as the blood moves back to the center of your body so you can do things like digest food, go to the bathroom, reactivate your immune system (especially to deal with any injuries you might have—I'll bet you pulled some muscles lifting that car off the ground!), and think logically again, too. Phew!

This all should work seamlessly to keep us alive, healthy, and balanced. The problem is that, in this day and age, people often feel stress all the time, and usually the source of that stress is abstract circumstances that we can't resolve simply with brute force. Even if it makes no sense to divert blood to your muscles when you are stressed about being able to pay your rent, that's what happens because, to your brain, stress is stress. And when you feel that feeling day in and day out for weeks and months and years on end, the parasympathetic system doesn't get its fair share of time. You're in fight, flight, or freeze mode almost constantly. This is chronic stress.

Chronic stress is a long-term response to an extended experience. Financial problems, relationship issues, trouble dealing with work, and the constant pressure to succeed, make more, do more, be more, be better, and win at life can all feel, to your body, like a life-or-death situation. In this scenario, the stress response isn't helping;

it's actually hurting. What you need when you can't pay your rent is to calm down and figure out a good solution, but that's not so easy when cortisol and adrenaline are misdirecting all your most valuable physical resources. This puts your body into an extreme physical state to the point of breaking down physically, mentally, and emotionally— because, of course, the beautiful, strong, resilient human body has its limits and just isn't made to be stressed out all the time.

Chronic stress will almost always cause other chronic problems over time. Just ask any doctor—90 percent of doctor's visits are for problems that are related to stress. Some symptoms of stress are vague and hard to pin down, like fatigue, irritability, depression, or problems with concentration and focus. Doctors don't really have an answer for those issues because they aren't diagnosable. They might send you home with some medication or just tell you to "relax." As if that's so easy to do! Stress can also result in situations like unhealthy weight loss or weight gain, extreme alcohol or drug use, or serious mental health issues, each of which have their own set of health consequences, from diabetes and heart attacks to fatty liver disease and debilitating addiction to self-harm. Stress is no joke.

Stress can even shrink your brain. My dear, you need your brain! According to the documentary *One Nation under Stress*,[2] chronic stress actually shrinks the prefrontal cortex, which is the part of the brain that manages our highest cognitive abilities. Over time, stress disconnects the circuits in this part of the brain, causing confusion, brain fog, and trouble concentrating. Over the long term, those circuits can atrophy and that part of the brain can literally waste away. At the same time, chronic stress seems to strengthen other parts of the brain—the ones that deal with emotional responses and impulsive behavior. This means that chronic stress can make you even less able to deal with life in a calm, objective way and more likely to react with uncontrolled emotion and impulsive responses, like violence and other irrational behaviors.

The very first thing you see in the documentary I just mentioned,

One Nation under Stress, is this statistic: "In the 1960s, Americans had among the highest life expectancy in the world. Today, the US ranks at the bottom of major developed nations." According to the experts in this documentary, for the first time ever, US life expectancy has dropped every year for three years in a row, and the main culprit—the "cause of the causes"—is stress. They attribute this drop in life expectancy to the huge number of premature deaths from what they call "deaths of despair"—drugs, alcohol, and suicide.

Even kids are feeling it—kids in the United States between the ages of fifteen and twenty-one say they experience frequent anxiety or depression from the threat of gun violence, rising suicide rates, worry about sexual harassment, and fear of being able to make enough money.[3] It's so sad that kids in high school and college have to be worried about these things. According to the researchers, this group has the worst mental health of any generation ever measured, with 27 percent reporting that their mental health was "fair" or "poor," and 91 percent saying they had experienced physical or emotional symptoms associated with stress, such as anxiety and depression. According to the Cigna U.S. Loneliness Index[4] survey of twenty thousand Americans, people between the ages of eighteen and thirty-seven are lonelier and claim to be in worse health than older generations. The beautiful children who will be running the world someday should be living carefree and happy lives, enjoying their youth, but as one teenager said in an interview (and I'm paraphrasing), how can you feel safe in the world if you can't even feel safe in school or at church?

I'm sure you can see why it is so important to intervene right now. The world we live in has a lot going on, which is why it is imperative to get our parasympathetic nervous systems to kick back in. This will help you to feel safe inside your body so that you can relax, slow down, and get aligned with your priorities.

Social media might be one of the biggest drivers of stress because so many of us spend so much time on social media sites. I certainly do—I love to post Instagram stories, record podcasts, and interact with people online, but I have had to learn my limits. The internet does a lot of good and can generate a feeling of community and connection, but about 45 percent of kids say social media makes them feel judged, while 38 percent say social media makes them feel bad about themselves. Online communication and social media exchanges are also so constant and incessant now that a lot of people never turn off. The first thing they do in the morning and the last thing they do at night is check their smartphones—and most Americans do it eighty times in between, or about every twelve minutes all day long. Most people start to feel anxious after ten minutes without looking at their phones and, in a recent study, when people were asked about some of the things they would rather do than lose their phones for just one day, 62 percent said they would rather go for a week without chocolate, 40 percent said they would rather lose their voice for an entire day, and 30 percent said they would rather give up sex for a week than go even one day without their phones! Among millennials, 88 percent sleep within reach of their phones, and most people in the study (of all ages), when asked how long they felt they could survive without their phones or food or water, assigned all three the same length of time: one day. More people check their phones when they wake up than kiss their spouses.[5]

We are always on call, expected to answer every text immediately so nobody ever thinks something is wrong or that we're slacking. Every ping distracts us, and shifts our attention away from what we're doing and toward our phones. Every "like" on Facebook or Instagram actually causes a shot of dopamine to the brain.[6] That sounds like an addiction to me.

FEAR CAUSES ANXIETY

In my work, one of the effects of stress I see the most is anxiety. My students tell me they have it. My clients tell me they have it. People in the audience when I speak come up to me afterward and tell me they have it.

I have the privilege of meeting with and speaking to large groups of people all over the world, so I've started asking them before they get a chance to tell me: "Do you experience anxiety?" During one of my keynote speeches to a group of seven hundred sorority girls at Penn State University, I asked them how many experienced anxiety at least weekly. Ninety percent raised their hands—and I suspect the other 10 percent were napping due to burnout!

These were mostly high-functioning, delightful, respectful, grateful, healthy girls, and yet they were feeling high levels of stress every day, not just about their schoolwork, but about their extracurricular activities and their personal lives. They were all constantly *doing*, and as they came up to talk to me after my speech, many of them shared their fear-based stories about how they were trying to get everything they could on their résumés so they could graduate as high achievers and get the right kind of job.

Most of these girls were around nineteen years old, yet they were feeling so much anxiety about who they were going to become, with zero faith and zero ability to trust in who they are right now. They looked like they had everything, but they were crumbling on the inside. They were coming up to me and crying, saying that it was the first time they had been given permission to feel their feelings and to consider that maybe they didn't have to walk around with all this stress. They had never realized that feeling differently is a choice.

Students aren't the only ones. I work with longtime successful businesspeople, running multimillion-dollar corporations, and when I ask them if they feel anxiety, they almost all say they struggle with it constantly. Ironically, women working in the wellness field seem to be especially prone to anxiety and overwhelm. Many of my colleagues are making magic in their industries, but almost all of them say they have anxiety or deep stress or burnout.

What is anxiety? The medical dictionary definition from Merriam-Webster says that anxiety is "an abnormal and overwhelming sense of apprehension and fear often marked by physical signs (such as tension, sweating, and increased pulse rate), by doubt concerning the reality and nature of the threat, and by self-doubt about one's capacity to cope with it."

In other words, unlike stress, which is a direct response to a directly threatening situation, anxiety is an indirect response—it is the fear that a directly threatening situation might happen, or happen again. When you can't pay a bill, you feel stress. When you fear getting the mail every day because you are afraid you will get a bill you can't pay, you feel anxiety. When you have to get up and give a speech, you feel stress. When you fear that you might have to get up and give a speech sometime during the semester or if you get promoted, you feel anxiety. If you lose your wallet or your passport, that's stressful. If you constantly feel your back pocket or dig through your purse to make sure you didn't lose your wallet or your passport, that's anxiety.

People express anxiety in different ways, so it doesn't always look the same. For some, it comes out as irritability, anger, sadness, depression, low self-esteem, loneliness, inability to get things done, or physical pain. In my case, anxiety caused severe back pain . . . and an addiction to Advil and alcohol. If you have anxiety, it might come in some completely different way, but in almost every case, I can say that anxiety is not caused by what is happening. It is caused by fear of what might happen or the inability to feel in control.

THE IMPORTANCE OF
MEDICATION AND/OR THERAPY

It's important to note that not all anxiety is based in your mind. If your biochemistry is imbalanced in any way, it can lead to a feeling of anxiety. I would never refute the biochemical basis of any mood disorder, which is why, when it comes to medication for chronic stress and/or mental health disorders such as anxiety or depression, sometimes this is the right answer. Medication can get you out of a place you can't get out of yourself by putting you in a state of more relaxed openness and clarity, so you can begin to look more deeply at what could be contributing to the problem. Traditional therapy can also help you work through the underlying triggers of your stress, burnout, anxiety, or depression. When the issue is resolved, you may no longer need the medication or therapy, but please always follow your doctor's advice.

You can still have anxiety—even if you have your health, even if you have a sense of purpose, even if you have a strong support network—as long as you aren't getting to the root of an old energy you never dealt with. A past event can imprint you with anxiety (I'll explain this more in the next chapter), and you can only defuse this kind of anxiety if you deal with the real source of your fear because anxiety masks feelings you don't want to feel or aren't ready to face.

Stress is normal and a necessary part of life, when it helps you rise to an occasion where you need to utilize your reserves for stressful life moments. However, when we are in a state of chronic stress, our bodies can feel that everything is a threat. This feeling of chronic stress that never subsides, and the anxiety that can spring out of this chronic stress state, is *not* a necessary part of life. Normal stress can help you survive in an emergency, or stay alert to things and get things done in your everyday life, but chronic stress and anxiety have no benefits.

They are purely destructive because they paralyze you, keep you from feeling free to live your life, and can harm you both mentally and physically. They can lead to health issues and they often lead to burnout.

Fortunately, there are potent remedies for chronic stress and anxiety. I'll talk more about how to work through these in the next two chapters.

BURNOUT COMES FROM PUSHING

Burnout is another complication of chronic stress. It's not the same as anxiety—it can *feel* more functional, because people often don't realize they have it, but, in reality, it's just as destructive. It might be easier to hide because you are still pushing yourself to keep on keeping on, but eventually you won't be able to maintain the façade. Burnout, like anxiety, is painful and you do not have to live with it.

Burnout is that feeling of not being able to do the basic things you need or want to do out of sheer exhaustion or loss of will, and it is caused by the belief that you need to constantly be doing, achieving, and being the best at everything you do, even when those efforts are wearing you out and making you unhappy. According to the World Health Organization (WHO), in its International Statistical Classification of Diseases and Related Health Problems, *burnout* is now considered a diagnosable syndrome that is "conceptualized as resulting from chronic workplace stress that has not been successfully managed."[7] The WHO lists the symptoms as feelings of energy depletion or exhaustion, increased mental distance from one's job or feelings of negativism or cynicism related to one's job, or reduced professional efficiency.

If you have been working too hard for too long, constantly hustling, grinding, and pushing yourself all the time because you think that is what you need to do to be successful, then you probably suffer from burnout. My father used to say that people spend the first part of their adulthood sacrificing their health to earn wealth, and they spend the second half of their adulthood spending their wealth to earn back their health.

If you have burnout, you might still be a super-high achiever, but when you get home from work, you feel unable to do even the easiest thing, like cook yourself a healthy dinner or go to a yoga class or joyfully engage with loved ones. You might be getting great performance reviews or have a flawless academic record, or your students or colleagues all think you are the best of the best, but inside you just want to crawl into bed and stay there for a year.

I've suffered from burnout many times in my life. There was even a time when I questioned if I should keep doing Reiki and the other work I do now because I had gotten so burned out. I was doing one-on-ones, I had a six-week waiting list for clients, I was doing retreats, I owned a fitness studio, I had a clothing line . . . it was too much. As much as I had already learned, I kept slipping back into that cycle of *more is more*. I kept pushing down those feelings of pressure, obligation, overwhelm, loneliness, guilt, and fear because I didn't think I had time to deal with them. Instead, I pretended that I didn't have deep feelings of self-dismissal. I was too over-obligated and while I was always there for my students and clients, I forgot to be there for myself. I was anxious, distant from my body, and burned out.

Burnout isn't always obvious to the people who have it because they are still so externally functional. When I was in the most stressful part of my life, with a high-pressure job in the US Senate, I didn't realize that I had burnout because I was doing so well at work. But the one clue was that I always felt overwhelmed. I would wake up every morning and feel a sense of extreme urgency before the day even started. I would be in a meeting or at lunch with someone and already thinking about what was coming next. I would be "relaxing" while thinking about everything else I needed to do, who I needed to call back that evening, what I had to take care of or wrap up or fix. That was burnout.

In the book *Burnout, Fatigue, Exhaustion,*[8] the authors pose a theory that periods in which many people in a population experience fatigue and feelings of burnout often happen after major social change. They see examples of this throughout history, such as after world wars, the industrial revolution, and rapid advances in technology. That certainly describes our world right now, as we are experiencing so many extreme events in the environment, in politics, and in relation to technology advancements and social violence. Social roles are changing fast, many people are in crisis, chronic diseases are at an all-time high, and it seems as if everybody is on edge.

Whether you identify most with the term *chronic stress, anxiety, burnout, overwhelm,* or just *fear,* stress is an underlying cause, and this book contains tools and practices to help you deal with it. Even though the autonomic nervous system operates without you directing it, you *can* influence it. You can stress yourself and turn on your sympathetic nervous system with nothing more than your thoughts, but, in the same way, you can also purposefully relax yourself and turn on your parasympathetic nervous system, and this is where our greatest opportunity to reset our system lies.

All the practices you will find in the last three chapters of this book have this effect (among many others). Chronic stress, anxiety, burnout, overwhelm, and fear are all signs from your body that you are not looking at something. Other signs are depression, grief, workaholism, isolation, disconnection, and lack of a clear life purpose. If you feel some of these things, this is your invitation to change that. Author Brené Brown said, "You either walk inside your story and own it, or you stand outside your story and hustle for your worthiness. You are imperfect, you are wired for struggle, but you are worthy of love and belonging." To burn bright is to walk inside your story with your entire self, embracing your imperfections and feeling your feelings and living your truth.

So let's take a look at your story.

~~~

CHAPTER TWO

Imprints: Your Pain Story

It is important to expect nothing, to take every experience, including the negative ones, as merely steps on the path, and to proceed.

—RAM DASS, AMERICAN SPIRITUAL LEADER AND AUTHOR

WITH GREAT LOVE and compassion, we're now going to move from what's happening in the world and how that external energy impacts stress and anxiety, to what is happening *in you*. We're going to look together, my love, with spaciousness and acceptance, at the feelings and emotions that have shaped you and influenced who and where you are right now in this present moment. When you see how you got here, you will be able to make a choice: to keep doing what you are doing to stay where you are, or to embrace change and all its gifts in order to shift into a life more in line with your true self.

THE POWER OF IMPRINTING

One of the most beautiful and the most painful things about humans is how much we *feel*. Since you were born (and maybe even before that in the womb), you have been having feelings. As you grew and had more experiences, good and bad, some of those experiences that caused strong feelings made imprints on you.

An imprint is a belief system or a deeply embedded memory that has altered how you see yourself, someone else, or the world. When something happens to you that leaves an impression, your central nervous system creates a picture of it and keeps it stored inside you. As it lives there, unprocessed, it can turn into what feels like an absolute truth, an unquestioned belief, an irrational fear, or, when the imprint is positive, a piece of wisdom, life guidance, or a positive self-concept. An imprint can make you act illogically, it can make you believe things that aren't true, and it can make you do things you wouldn't otherwise do. That's because imprints aren't based on your current reality. They come from a past moment or a past reality (or your perception of a past reality). You can grow out of them, but if you hang on to them, they keep you acting from a place that may no longer be relevant for your life. They can hold you back from growth and stepping into the now of your life.

Imagine two people walking down the street together at night. They are both in exactly the same environment and are both at exactly the same risk of danger, whatever that may be. Yet, one of them feels safe because, as a child, she got a lot of attention and reassurance and is imprinted with a feeling of security. The other doesn't feel safe because, as a child, he was often put in precarious situations and he didn't feel protected, so he was imprinted with a sense that life is dangerous. Maybe these two people were safe and maybe they were in danger, but neither one of them is perceiving the present moment because they are both operating under the influence of imprints.

When you respond to the right-now based on the before, you

cannot ever really exist in the right-now. Your vision of reality will always be clouded by your imprints. This could be happening to you in this moment. Imprints may be affecting how you deal (or don't deal) with what happens to you in life, how you think about things, and how you see yourself when you look in the mirror. Imprints are most deeply formed in childhood, but you can keep accumulating them throughout your entire life. With every imprint, your response to your own feelings will shift and your interaction with your feelings will get more complicated. That's being human, and it's okay. If, as a child, you touched a stovetop and it was hot, you made an imprint to help you avoid hurting yourself in the future. We are all shaped by stories from our past and labels that we've put on ourselves, or that others have tagged us with. Imprints will always be with us, but what we can do to decrease their power is to become aware of them.

Now, my dear, think back to your earliest memories, when you were just a few years old. Of all the trillions of impressions you have taken in throughout your childhood, some have stuck with you over others. The memories you still hold on to and think about are clues to your imprints. What can you remember about the things that have formed your beliefs about life and yourself? You may not have early memories, and that's okay. Just try to identify a time or a moment in your life, when you were younger, when a belief or a thought became ingrained in you. Just pick one. Maybe your family labeled you as "the smart one" or "the outgoing one" or "the introvert." Maybe in school, you felt like "the loner" or "popular" or "too sensitive" or "the best violin player in school." Maybe you thought of yourself as "clumsy" or "bookish" or "rebellious." It could be a good imprint or perhaps a sad one. Think about it and see if you can feel the feeling you had when the imprint was made, but bring your adult awareness and the knowledge you have now to the feeling you had then.

This is the beginning of awareness that can bring your imprints into the light where you can become conscious of them and release their control over you. Identifying and re-feeling these early memories can help point you to the labels you have put on yourself and the stories you believe about yourself or others. You may still be imprinted with the idea that you were "a difficult toddler" or "the star of the school play" or that you "can't sit still" or that you "have great hair" or that you are "the shy one" or "the loud one" or "never enough." Some of these imprints may seem trivial, but they can all influence your perception of life in ways that put a layer between you and your truth, your value, and your reality in this present moment. Just hold this intention of becoming aware of your imprints in your heart and see what arises over the next few days as you open yourself to recalling these early experiences. Please try to get radically curious, and maybe even journal out a few things that arise.

✦ THE TRIAD OF BODY, MIND, AND SPIRIT ✦

The body, the mind, and the spirit interact with all parts of life—with pain, with joy, with health, with relationships, and with awareness. Each of these things can have a physical, mental, or spiritual manifestation, and each of these is tied to the others, in a triad, like this:

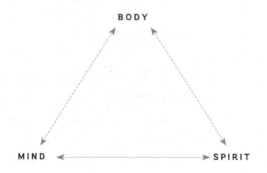

I'll talk more about this triad in chapter 4, but it has always been at the core of my teaching. Throughout this book, I will keep referring back to this triad and the way each part connects with every other part, so keep this in mind as we talk about imprints and the effects they can have on people.

As you explore what you believe to be true about yourself, you will begin to recognize where those beliefs originated, and you will be able to bring into clearer focus whether they are actually true, or still feel true. In many cases, if not most, old imprints (especially negative ones) were never really true, or are no longer true, beyond the ways in which you have made them true in your own life because of your belief in them. For example, if you believe you aren't smart, the truth is not that you aren't smart. The truth is that *you believe you aren't smart*, and that could have affected how you have lived your life up until now. To help you unpack this idea, let's look at some examples of imprints in some of my clients, students, friends, and fellow teachers. Some of their examples may resonate with you or bring up things for you that you thought you had forgotten.

〰〰〰

SOFT IMPRINTS

Soft imprints are the beliefs you have that may not seem on the surface to be all that important, but they can still hold you back from the recognition of your fullness and value. Soft imprints hurt a little bit, but you can usually shake them off or make excuses for them. They feel like minor imperfections—they are emotionally cosmetic, but they can last for years. They are like scratches on the surface of your personality. They often take the form of bad habits, or mild insecurities, or urges that you follow without really thinking about them.

One of the soft imprints I carried for years was about my voice. I have a vivid memory of trying out for the school choir in elementary school. I didn't make the cut, and I was devastated. Out of shame for this "failure," I told the music teacher that I had a cold and that was why I didn't sing well. I didn't have a cold. I knew I didn't sound good, but I felt that I needed to make an excuse for my failure. My dad was a wonderful singer and I loved singing, too. It was something we had in common, or so I thought. It had never occurred to me that I might not be good at it but, after that experience, I stopped singing for years. In church, my parents would pinch me and nudge me to sing along to the hymns, but I was afraid of my own voice. I had labeled myself as a "bad singer," even though nobody had actually told me I was a *bad* singer. The only thing that really happened is that I wasn't chosen for the school choir—nobody ever said I should stop trying.

But I lived with that label for decades. It wasn't until much later, when I started doing healing work, that I dared to sing when I was alone in the car. I let all the crackling, off-key sounds come out and, at first, I judged myself. I sounded terrible! But since nobody else was judging me, I kept doing it, always when I was alone. After a while, my voice began to improve. I was practicing, playing with the sound, and it was helping. I gained confidence. Sometimes I would cry in the car as the new sounds came out of my body—it was such a release and a relief. The more I sang, the better it sounded and the more free I felt.

I wasted years of my life not doing something I loved, all because of an imprint. It turns out that label wasn't true at all. I *can* sing. I'm not going to quit my day job and go on the road or anything, but singing brings me joy now, and I'm so glad I was able to find it again and discover that sound could be more than joyful for me—it could be a therapy. Sometimes I use sound just to loosen up and shake up stuck feelings. You can empty the energy of the body through the vibration of sound. At other times, when I'm feeling overwhelmed or stuck or in pain, I'll start to release sound without any thought of what it would sound like to someone else. It might come out as a song, but it might just be a fluttering of my lips or sticking my tongue out with a big exhale and opening my jaw and releasing. I love to do this in my car— I'll make all sorts of noises. Try this when you are alone and feel the energy moving inside you. Make any noise that feels good and imagine that you are freeing something inside yourself that you have been holding on to. Surrender to the sound!

Jen is a fellow Reiki teacher who had a similar experience, but for her, it was in math. When she was nine years old, her math teacher took her aside at recess and, while literally looking down at her, said, "Jenny, you are terrible at math. You should *not* keep going with it." Jen still remembers exactly where she was standing, where the teacher was standing, and exactly how the teacher's face looked when she said this. She remembers thinking, "How can I not keep going with math? I still have to go to math class."

For years afterward, Jen believed she was bad at math, bad with numbers, and bad with money, all because of the imprint formed by that one comment from that one teacher. It wasn't until she began to learn about numerology and began to operate her own successful business as a massage therapist, Reiki master and teacher, and life coach, that she realized she was actually pretty good with numbers and was able to manage the financial aspects of her business with no problem. She told me that now she looks back at that poor little Jenny she once was and sends her love and compassion.

Another one of my personal soft imprints was about conformity. When I was in junior high, I remember the kids in my class all decided that leather jackets were cool, and suddenly we all absolutely had to have leather jackets. Did I like leather jackets? Not particularly. But when everyone else decided we should all love them, I decided I had to love them, too. I was at an impressionable age when friends felt like the most important thing in the world, so I went along with this fad, and reinforced my own inner feeling that it was important to be accepted by the group. Whether it's leather jackets in junior high or hot yoga in your thirties, conformity isn't necessarily bad. It's a natural human tendency. But when conformity becomes an imprint that gets in the way of your own self-alignment, it can become harmful. It's one thing to think, "That leather jacket looks cool. I think I'll get one, too," or "Hot yoga sounds interesting. I think I'll try it." But when conformity has become imprinted, it will feel more like, "Everybody has a leather jacket. If I don't have one, I won't be as good as everybody else," or "Hot yoga makes me want to pass out, but I have to keep going because all my friends are doing it."

Comparison is another soft imprint reinforced in this digital age because we all have the opportunity to compare ourselves to other people hundreds of times a day on social media. Take my teenage leather jacket years and my thirteen-year-old deep desire to fit in and "be cool," then increase those desires exponentially. Instead of wanting to fit in with a small cohort of school friends, thirteen-year-olds now have millions of people to compare themselves to, as they see the highlights of their lives in front of them all day long. Can you imagine the number of imprints caused by those micro-subconscious comparison moments as kids (and adults) scroll through their feeds every day? Social media can continue to imprint us well into adulthood.

I see conformity imprints playing out in my fellow teachers and clients all the time. Many people who are business owners, teachers, or supervisors want their teams or students or clients to like them and they want to feel that they are one of the group, rather than being the teacher or the leader. Conformity imprints could also be the reason that groups of friends over time tend to all end up with similar qualities, have the same opinions, and even the same marital status— married couples tend to stay married or are more likely to get divorced, depending on what their friends are doing.[1]

Soft imprints can turn into profound imprints if you don't surround them with awareness. The next time you tell yourself you can't do something, or aren't good at something, or have to do something because everyone else is doing it, ask yourself: Do *I* really want that thing, support that action, believe that idea? What do *I* really think? What do *I* really want? Is this really *me*? Maybe you aren't sure of the answer right away, but if you give yourself permission to consider whether your first impulse is right and in harmony with your true desire *today*, you may discover an imprint. You may suddenly recognize that your urge to buy that handbag, or apologize all the time, or eat out of boredom, or gossip to your friends, or whatever it is, doesn't feel quite as compelling anymore, just because you looked directly at those feelings, got radically curious about your beliefs, and saw where they were really coming from.

~~~~

PROFOUND IMPRINTS

Profound imprints are imprints that go deeper. Soft imprints land on your body and cross your mind, but profound imprints get inside your body and burrow deep inside your mind. Profound imprints are things like fear of loss/abandonment, fear of commitment, poverty consciousness, the drive to push constantly, and the fear of failure/ success. These imprints can last a lifetime, and they can come from traumatic events, or from reinforcement over a long period, such as throughout an entire childhood. They hold you back from the full expression of your you-ness. If soft imprints are scratches, profound imprints are wounds that can leave scars on the body, the mind, or the spirit.

Here's an example of a profound imprint that lands in the body. Anne is a colleague of mine who will never forget her first day of kindergarten, when she sat on the seesaw on the playground. She was always the tallest girl in the classroom, but she wasn't self-conscious about it. A fifth-grade girl climbed onto the other end of the seesaw and the seesaw didn't move. The girl yelled so all the kids could hear: "That kindergarten kid is heavier than a fifth-grader!" Anne was mortified! It was the first time she ever felt embarrassed about her body. Even today, she struggles with feeling "too big" when that old imprint gets triggered. When she thinks she weighs too much or feels taller than everyone or even when she "acts too big" by talking too loudly or getting too much attention, she struggles with shame. "Too big" is her imprint. She used to think that when she "got smaller," like after dieting, she was more worthy. It wasn't until she began a regular meditation practice (page 162) and began to manage moments of body anxiety with tapping (page 167) that she finally began to see that she is beautiful and worthy of love just as she is, no matter what size she is or what confidence level she has at any given moment. It has changed her entire life and level of happiness.

My friend Jenna is another good example. When she was young, her parents told her that she had some learning disabilities. Jenna was a daydreamer in school and she had a hard time staying focused on things that didn't interest her. She was put into the "slow reading group" (she was the only girl) because sometimes she had to reread things a few times to comprehend them. Throughout her adult life, she has struggled with the imprint that she isn't smart. Even though her reading trouble was in grade school and has long since been resolved, she has moments of doubt in her abilities, or thinks she isn't good enough. Even in her very successful career of twenty-five years, during which she has been consistently promoted, she has moments of thinking she is failing or not being effective in her work. She has come a long way working on this imprint. Meditation has helped her see this as something that is no longer true (and may have never been true), and she is now aware of when this imprint comes up in her mind. But it's still there, and she often has to remind herself that just because something goes wrong at work does not mean there is anything wrong with *her*.

Another example of a profound imprint that lands in the spirit energy is my client Amy. Amy is a middle child. Her older sister was creative, dramatic, and talented at singing, acting, dancing, and getting all the attention. Amy loved music and drama, but she was a quieter person and she felt so outdone by her big sister that she turned away from the things she loved and focused all her energy on the two things her older sister wasn't good at: math and sports. Also, because her sister was so social, Amy felt like she couldn't compete in that area, so she became more withdrawn and less willing to reach out for connection with others. In sports, she played tennis because she could play without constant interaction with a team, and she got a degree in accounting and works for herself so she doesn't have to interact with work colleagues very often. It wasn't until she was in her forties that she realized she really loved to teach. She began coaching kids in tennis and homeschooling her kids, and she felt much more like herself.

I still struggle with my own profound imprints. When I was young, my parents were stressed a lot of the time. My dad was the director of physical therapy at a hospital and had a private practice, and my mother was a drug and alcohol counselor, working on her PhD. They were both busy with their jobs, constantly trying to make ends meet, and because my sister is nine years older than I am and my brother is nine years younger, they were raising kids for thirty-six years. They were both workaholics and they both had substance abuse problems, too. On top of all that, my mother had been diagnosed with severe depression and sometimes had to be hospitalized.

My parents were very accomplished people, and I learned from an early age that work equaled worthiness. How hard you worked determined your value. My mom especially was always doing something. She rarely just sat down on the couch to watch an entire TV program. Usually, she was working or studying, baking or cleaning, or doing *something*—always doing something. She was the oldest of seven children, so she was imprinted herself, at an early age, with the idea that she had to be responsible for everyone. She once told me that, as a teenager, she had a date with the young man who would become my father, and her mother (my grandmother) handed her a big basket of laundry and told her she wasn't going anywhere until it was all cleaned and pressed. So even as an adult and a mother herself, she was operating under the imprint that she had to be constantly *doing* to matter, to have permission for things, and to be of value.

When I was in high school, my mom had to have ECT treatments (electroconvulsive therapy, once known as "shock treatment") for her depression. Sometimes she couldn't remember things that happened the week before because of the treatments, which apply electricity to the brain. But even going through all that, she never stopped going to work. Unless she actually had to leave us for weeks at a time to check into a facility, she never gave herself any time to just rest and recover. I am in awe of her ability to keep going through so much mental and physical pain, but I don't think it was healthy for her or for our family. The imprint stamped into me throughout all the years of my childhood was this: *No matter what is wrong with you, you have to keep going, keep working, keep showing up and showing everybody that you are okay, capable, and reliable. Even when you feel as if you're going to break, you still need to show up. Push your emotions down and keep going.*

But being so busy with work and her own mental health issues, my mom didn't have much left inside her to take care of me consistently, or at least that was my perception—that she could barely take care of herself at times. Her doing was all externally focused. I sensed this at a very young age, and realized that I was better off taking care of myself. I didn't want to be a burden on my busy parents, so I became obsessed with self-sufficiency. I got myself rides to many of my extracurricular activities, signed up for things myself, and figured most of it out on my own—homework, permission slips, lunches, socializing. I started babysitting at a young age and earning as much money as I could, and I hoarded it like a miser. My first job was at a Subway sandwich shop when I was fourteen years old, and I remember being so proud to be a sandwich artist that I dreamed about it the night before. I wanted to *do*. That's what drove me. It was empowering, but I was also operating under the imprint that I would achieve worthiness through doing, doing, doing. And all this doing was for me (and probably for my mother) a way of avoiding feeling the feelings that would terrify me if I really looked at them.

Nobody in my extended family talked about my mother's mental illness. We lived in a small city in North Dakota, and it was an unspoken rule in my family that when it came to our personal problems, they were nobody's business. I learned early on that you weren't supposed to talk about your emotions. I felt like there wasn't usually any space in our home to talk about things in a real, open, and supportive way. We just had to keep going and pretending there was nothing wrong. Even my best friend since age five had no idea that my mom suffered from depression. When we were older and in our thirties, I finally started to share some of the stories, and she was in disbelief that she had never known or even suspected what was going on in my family.

My mom's side of the family was incredibly fun and loving, and we had many wonderful moments all together as a family. But this was confusing for me because this whole side of the family was also prone to drama and teasing and getting angry about teasing. If things were good, we had a great time, but nobody was sympathetic to any real, deep feelings. You had to be able to take a joke, even if it was a mean-spirited joke. It took me a long time to realize that ridiculing someone and preying on their insecurities and fears was not an expression of love—that imprint caused me a lot of pain in relationships and questions about my self-worth that took me a long time to get over.

The imprints that come from family can be the most influential of all. Profound imprints can influence you throughout your life—when you get your first job, when you find someone you love, when you choose how you dress, what you feel most passionate about, how you talk to other people, and what you see when you look in the mirror. The belief system you have tells you how things in your life will go, directs you in how to approach things, and tells you what you can and can't do, and what is acceptable or unacceptable for others to do to you. Even with all the work I've done to overcome my tendency to prioritize productivity over self-reflection and to push myself too hard, I still struggle with it and slip back into my old patterns sometimes: workaholism, denial, anxicty, self-deprecation, and holding in the pain.

The way to bring awareness to your imprints is to explore all the places in your body, mind, and spirit where you feel a disharmony. Maybe you can't stand to look at a certain part of your body. That could be because of an imprint. Maybe you are afraid of particular kinds of food. That could be an imprint. Maybe you have social anxiety and dread going to events where you know there will be a lot of people. Maybe you obsess about work all the time, but you don't feel truly engaged, empowered, or interested in your work. Maybe you carefully control everything you eat and exercise religiously, but you still feel unhealthy or insecure about your body. Maybe people have always told you that you are good at something, but deep down, you don't want to do that thing. Or people have always told you that you are bad at something, but you long to do that thing. These are disharmonies. When you don't feel free or at ease and something feels off, these are clues to imprints. At some level inside yourself, you know that you should care for and love your body, that it's okay to enjoy food, that socializing at your will is heathy, and that work can be in balance with other parts of your life. Some part of you knows that it's not healthy to obsess about things or to neglect them completely, and that it's healthy to follow your passions. Some part of you knows that you know yourself better than anyone else knows you. The imprints that caused these feelings of imbalance may not be immediately obvious to you, but expand your awareness and leave the question open: Why do I feel this disharmony? Where does this discomfort originate? Where do I feel imbalanced? Why do I do this, even though I know it is not in my best interest? Open the door for insights, breathe through the thoughts and discomforts, and wait for the imprints to become apparent to you.

WHEN IMPRINTS TURN PHYSICAL

It's quite common for unacknowledged imprints to surface as physical pain. It's so much easier to say "My back is killing me!" than it is to say "I'm terrified that my mom might commit suicide" or "I'm terrified that I might be impossible to love."

This is what happened to me. After graduation, I got my first job as a legislative correspondent in the US Senate, on Capitol Hill in Washington, DC. This was the perfect job to fuel my workaholism, but even that wasn't enough for me. Whenever I was faced with alone time, I got panicky and took on more *doing*. Being alone, where I might have the chance to think about my feelings for a minute, was too terrifying, so I started babysitting again, I got a job at a bar, I joined a dance company, and I taught dance classes.

Sometimes I would feel anxious for no apparent reason, but I never faced that feeling. I just pushed it down and kept going. I will never forget the time my mother called me at work from the psych ward. She was yelling and saying crazy things to me—I was terrified that she might be in a psychotic state. I had to pretend that everything was normal because I was sitting there at my desk, surrounded by people, but my heart was racing and my mind was spiraling. After I hung up, I went to the bathroom and broke down, sobbing. But then I took a few deep breaths, washed my face, and went back to work. I didn't tell anyone. All I could do was tell myself, over and over again, "Keep going. You're okay. You're good." I wasn't okay, but if I said it enough, I could kind of convince myself.

Then the back pain started. There was no obvious cause. It was in the middle of my back, on the left side, and I don't think it was a coincidence that it was right behind my heart. At first the pain was nagging, then it became excruciating, then debilitating. I started popping Advil all day long, and at night I would kill the pain with red wine and more Advil just to be able to sleep.

It was also no coincidence that, at the time, I was involved in a toxic relationship with a manipulative boyfriend and felt like I couldn't get away. Whenever I broke up with him, he would manage to get me to come back. During the summer, I had broken up with him and took a backpacking trip to Europe with a girlfriend, and when I got back, my ex-boyfriend convinced me to come over. We slept together and I spent the night. The next morning, while I was brushing my teeth, suddenly the whole right side of my neck froze.

This was the most pain I had ever experienced. I couldn't move my head. I couldn't stand or sit without searing pain. I tried to ignore it. That night, I had to work at the bar, and instead of going to the emergency room, I did the only thing I knew how to do—keep showing up and doing. I went to work my bar shift and within about two hours, I was lying flat on a bench, unable to move without extreme pain. My ex-boyfriend met me at the emergency room (one of the only times I recall him doing a semi-selfless act), where they diagnosed me with a bulging disk. They gave me a cortisone shot and some pain meds, and they put me in a neck brace.

This was one of the lowest points in my life. I was exhausted, overwhelmed, and spiraling downward. Everything in my life felt as out of place as my neck. Then I got diagnosed with mono. My immune system was shot. I had been sick almost every month that year with something or other. I was regularly taking antibiotics, I had several urinary tract infections (UTIs), and at one point I was even on steroids. I felt as if there were no way out. I was trapped inside my own life, trapped in my relationship, trapped in my five jobs, trapped in my malfunctioning body. I knew it was just a matter of time before the next terrible thing happened, but I wasn't even scared anymore. I had accepted that this was my life and nothing would ever change.

One afternoon, I was lying on my ex-boyfriend's couch, crying after another one of our big fights that left me feeling crazy, insecure, and unloved, when the phone rang. It was a friend of mine who lived in New York. She told me that she was moving to Los Angeles to pursue her acting career. She said, "You're miserable, Kels. You should come with me."

My first thought was that of course I couldn't do something like that. Leave all my jobs and just take off for Los Angeles? It was crazy, right? But a little part of me felt a door opening, and, within minutes, I realized I had to take this chance. Even though I was terrified, I knew that if I stayed in Washington, DC, I would never find peace or escape the cycle of on-again-off-again with my ex-boyfriend. This was my opportunity to change my life. It was right there in front of me. All I had to do was say yes. My emotional strength was as thin as a thread, but on that tiny filament of self-love, I made a choice.

Sometimes, a drastic change can break the spell of a profound imprint. Although moving to Los Angeles didn't immediately resolve all those deep imprints, it broke me out of a place I didn't think I could escape. That shook me out of my self-destructive loop and allowed me to start shifting and looking at my life in a new way. Of course, the first thing I did when I got to LA was to find another high-pressure job, this time for a Fortune 500 company, but I also felt like I had more time and space to focus on finally healing my back pain. I began to surround myself with supportive people, and I began to see other people practicing self-care, which made me think that maybe it was okay for me to do that, too. After a couple of years of living there, I found myself surrounded by people committed to eating healthy food, being outside, taking yoga classes, and healing themselves. Step by step I began to follow their cues, not because of comparison or conformity, but because they looked peaceful, healthy, and happy in their lives, and I wanted to feel that way, too.

The first thing I tried was yoga. I had done some hot yoga in college, but I really didn't think it was my thing. In LA, though, everyone was doing it, so I decided to give it another try, and went to a yoga class with a friend. (This is one instance where conformity served me.) After the class, I was lying on my mat in savasana ("corpse pose"), and I felt a strange, startling sensation in my chest, as if my heart were literally shifting or shaking loose inside me. You know that feeling you get when a big truck rumbles by and it shakes the ground or the building you're in? It was like that, but there was no truck. I'd never felt anything like that before. I asked my friend about it. She just shrugged and said, "That's why people do yoga."

Within just a few weeks of regular classes, I noticed that my back didn't hurt quite as much as before and my anxiety had dissipated. I didn't think it could possibly be the yoga. After that initial heart shift, yoga didn't seem to be doing anything at all. But I couldn't deny that I had less pain. I also realized that I felt a bit clearer, and I had a little more energy. I still hadn't recognized that I had a castle full of stress in my body that had never been opened. Now I know that my body and my energy were changing because yoga was helping me release some stress, but, at the time, I only knew I wanted more of whatever I was getting.

Fast-forward to a few years later. I had gained a lot of weight from traveling almost every week for my corporate job, so I thought maybe I needed to exercise more. I started to get into a new fitness method called Pure Barre. After just a few weeks of taking classes, I was asked to start teaching. As a former dancer, it brought me so much joy to be moving and holding a ballet barre again. Teaching was an even bigger joy for me. Just after I started to train to become a Pure Barre instructor, I met the man who would become my husband, and, within a year, he convinced me to open my own Pure Barre studio. I made the leap with a friend—ours was the first Pure Barre studio in Beverly Hills, and just the second or third one in Los Angeles. One evening, I created a wellness night at the studio for clients, and a friend who was an aesthetician asked if she could bring a Reiki healer to do mini healing sessions at the wellness event.

Reiki? Never heard of it. When I learned what it was, I thought it sounded kind of ridiculous. How could you heal people if you weren't even touching them? It didn't make any sense to me, and I was totally skeptical that it would do anything, but my clients seemed interested. When the healer invited me to do a free session with her, as a thank-you for inviting her to the event, I supposed it couldn't hurt. I was always willing to try something new. By that time, I had tried several different kinds of healing techniques in LA for the sake of my back pain, so why not one more?

She performed Reiki and EFT (emotional freedom technique, or tapping) on me, and, afterward, I was astonished. My pain wasn't entirely gone, but it had dissipated significantly. More than anything else, I hadn't felt that peaceful in years . . . if ever!

I began to see this Reiki practitioner regularly, and after several months of weekly sessions, I decided I wanted to learn how to do it on myself. I took her Reiki Level 1 training. Then I got braver. I started moving more outside my box. I went on some yoga retreats. I did some workshops. And, slowly but surely, my body continued to shift and my mind began to calm down. My workaholism became less appealing; the addictive call of caffeine highs and red wine "relaxation" became less tempting. I felt as if my chronic pain was slowly burning away.

But it wasn't just my pain that was changing. I was changing. I was becoming more confident. I began to feel that maybe I was enough, just as me. I began to believe that I could accomplish and create the things I desired. I began to feel calm and in the present moment, and I began to be okay not doing something every moment. Going inward began to feel more natural, and I started to understand that perhaps my physical pain was linked to my emotional pain, and if I dealt with one, it might naturally support the other. I was becoming more self-aware.

The better I felt about myself and the more I questioned the stories I'd told myself about who I was, the more I grew and the less I hurt. I became a Reiki master, a meditation teacher, and a yoga instructor, and now I travel all over the world, teaching, leading retreats, giving lectures, and helping other people free themselves from their own physical, mental, and emotional blocks. I am living in much greater harmony with who I really am than I ever have before, and my back hardly ever hurts anymore.

A decade ago, I could not have imagined that I would ever have the life I have now, and I probably wouldn't be here today if I had never questioned who I was, how I was living, and what was really true about the limits on my ability to live a life filled with ease and flow and immense amounts of joy. I had to accept that my back pain wouldn't resolve until I accepted responsibility for the feelings I was afraid to feel. When I was finally able to do that, the pain began to subside.

My story isn't unique. I have had thousands of students and clients with similar stories about physical pain or health issues caused by the denial of emotions and the refusal to feel feelings. Like my student Cam, who never felt that she had a voice in her family and now, every time she is stressed, has terrible neck and throat pain. And my friend Greta, who moved fourteen times during grade school and now has chronic pain in her lower back whenever she feels unsafe and ungrounded. And my client Janine, who has always had to carry the weight of her mentally ill younger sister on her shoulders and suffers from literal shoulder pain every day. Every one of them found relief using techniques in this book.

What I want you to know is that if any of these stories resonate with you, you can give yourself permission to look at your pain. You can surround it with awareness to feel what it might mean and where it started. Sometimes, all you need to do to shake up your old pattern and make things look different is to do something different. You don't need to move across the country (although maybe that would be right for you). It might just mean you eat in a different way for a while, or move in a different way for a while, or go somewhere new. Meet someone new. Try something new. Ask for help. Take a nap in the middle of the day. Talk about what's going on. Write about how you feel. Work out when you feel like napping. Stop trying so hard to hold on to a life that isn't working. Get ready to become radically curious about your life.

There is healing available for you. It doesn't have to take the years it took for me to figure out this connection. You can begin healing your own pain—whatever kind of pain it is—right now. All you have to do, my dear, is let yourself feel.

✦ TRIPLE-A MOMENT ✦

We all need help sometimes. We all need support. When your car breaks down, you get a flat tire, or you run out of gas, you can call AAA, the motor club. But when you break down, when your "tires" are flat, you're out of "gas," you've locked your proverbial keys in the car, and you've lost your center and feel overwhelmed, stop what you are doing and take a Triple-A moment. Ask yourself these three questions:

Aware: What do I not want to be aware of or feel in this moment?

Accept: What am I refusing to accept about myself in this moment?

Action: What action can I take to support myself in this moment?

The answers can direct you toward exactly what you can choose to be aware of and feel, what you can choose to accept, and what you can choose to act upon, to break out of your sense of overwhelm and regain your balance and power.

MASTERING CHANGE

Think about what scares you—think about the things you dream of, the things that you don't really believe you can have so you push them away. Those things are your nectar. Those things are your medicine, and no matter how far away they seem, everything you need to achieve them is already inside you. You have everything you need, so you don't have to fear. What scares you is where the answers are, where the action is.

When you are triggered by that thing you fear, just notice its presence inside you. You don't have to do anything extreme. Just make a mental note: "There's that thing again that I'm trying so hard not to see." Is it real? Or is it just fear? People sometimes make fear into an acronym: FEAR—False Evidence Appearing Real. That's what fear is usually based on—false evidence.

Sure, it's easier to do what you've always done, even if it isn't good for you, than to make a big change. Change may be scary, but to keep chasing only what you know or to stay in your comfort zone forever is to go in circles, like a dog chasing its tail. When you go in circles, nothing changes. But if you stop running those old programs and letting your imprints control your life, when you make a choice to do something differently, you will see a whole new universe of possibility for your life.

The voice of fear inside you may be there right now, and maybe it will always be there, but, as with a radio, you get to decide how loud the volume goes. You are the master of your fear. A dog doesn't walk around tail-first. The tail is an afterthought. Your fear can inform you when you need to be careful, but it never, ever has to be your boss. Don't walk around fear-first. You can live led by your brightness, not by your darkness.

Too much "safe" keeps you disconnected from your soul. To change is to grow, to embrace new awareness, and to be willing to see other possibilities than the ones that have kept you in a rut or in a thought spiral or in anxiety, burnout, or overwhelm. Also, change is inevitable anyway. Everything changes. Everything cycles and fluctuates. You can't control it. There is no safety in staying the same because you can't stay the same. Staying the same is just denial. Change is going to happen, whether you decide to flow with it or you decide to fight it. The truth is, you don't actually know what change will bring to your life. It could bring something more amazing, healthful, joyful, creative, peaceful, or supportive than what you have right now.

Or maybe change will bring some difficulty for a while. That's okay. In every difficulty, in every challenge, is an opportunity to grow. Whatever happens, you are right on time. You are okay. Flow with it, feel it, be willing to move with it, and things will work out. The only thing you can know for sure is that change is coming, so you might as well accept that and work on knowing yourself better so you can experience the changes you really want deep inside. You wouldn't be reading this book if you weren't seeking some kind of change. Don't miss the opportunities that present themselves to you because you are afraid to receive them.

Will you choose fear? Or will you choose love? Just imagine what your life would look like if fear had nothing to do with the way you live your life and be you. What would your life look like if you acted according to your desires and dreams, *in spite of fear*? What would your life look like if you embraced change as the path to your true self and a life of harmony and joy? You would light up the world.

~~~~~

BE BIG, BE BRIGHT

When you recognize and come to terms with your own pain story, as it has manifested in a physical, mental, or spiritual way, you will find your inner power to override those programs and step into who you are right here and now, unburdened by labels and stories that don't serve you.

For years, I thought something was wrong with me. I was a victim of self-imposed smallness. I was so unaware of what I was doing to myself that I thought my feelings of not being enough were a symptom of something wrong with me. I thought I was wrong to have such big desires and dreams. Instead of embracing my secret desires and my brightness and my desire to live a life of purpose, of inspiration, of joy, and of sharing, I felt constant shame. I tried everything not to be that person who was big and bright—I tried to make myself small. That is how I made myself suffer—oh, so much more than was necessary! I wasn't giving myself permission to be fully myself—to be wild, free, and uninhibited.

I still feel stressed sometimes, and I can still experience pain and anxiety, but now I have the tools to lean into it, and the context in which to more fully understand what it is. When I ignore my own needs, when I let the stress get to me, the first place I always feel it is in my back, right behind my heart. Those twinges of pain are reminders that I need to get back inside my body. They are fingers pointing to my heart and saying, "Go back to square one. Get back to you. Square one is right here."

When you let yourself inhabit your fullness, aligning your external environment with your internal reality, you will expand into whatever amount of space you have created for yourself, internally and externally. For some people, that may mean expanding their external energy, as I needed to do; for others, it might mean becoming quieter, more introspective, or even retreating somewhat on the outside in order to explore and grow and expand on the inside.

When you take all the space you need, you will experience ease. When you dare to bring awareness to your situation, you do a trust fall backward into a joyful life. This is what your soul has been waiting and longing for: the cure rising up from inside your own being. The minute you start trusting yourself and your truth, you will feel a shift. That may mean instituting a new practice, setting up a boundary, turning in a new direction, even getting out of a relationship or quitting your job. Whatever it is, keep nurturing that awareness, and eventually you will know what to do.

There is a flame inside each one of us. If you are alive, there is a flame inside you, even if it's just the tiniest spark keeping you alive right now. If you are lying on the couch in rest-digest-repair mode, you can be in your brightness. If you are out in the world shining and giving and doing and burning, showing everybody what you have to offer, you can be in your brightness. Sometimes you may feel intense and electric energy. Sometimes you may feel cool and calm energy. But if you nourish your inner flame, you can always be in your brightness, even if you feel dark and stuck.

There is nothing wrong with pain. Pain is a teacher. We all have our light and we all have our darkness, and light is easiest to see and acknowledge in the dark. Your brightness is brighter because you have been through darkness. A city is brightest at night. A candle is most illuminating in the shadows.

A teacher once told me that if someone is down in a pit of darkness and you are standing above in the light, looking down, you can't help the person in the dark by going down into the darkness with them. Instead, you can stay standing in the light so that the person can see the light from the darkness, and can choose to climb up into the light when they are ready.

If you are the light in the darkness, others can see how to come into the light. And if you are the one who is in the darkness, you can know there is light coming from what you are experiencing. Walking your own path in your truth will bring you to your own light, which, in turn, lights the way for others, and this is how you can bring more goodness into the world. People may judge you, get mad at you, project labels onto you, try to imprint you, but, ultimately, when you burn bright, nothing will dim your flame. You are who you are, no matter what's going on around you. You can choose to trust it and know it.

Your goal is not to erase or deny your shadows, but to face them, pull them apart, and examine them to find the truths inside them. Imprints are always with us, and no matter how much progress we have made, there are always times when we go out into the world and subconsciously put ourselves into situations that will reconfirm our imprints. But when you bring awareness to those hidden parts of yourself, you can dismantle your pain story and discover who's really in there. When you pull up the rug of your fear and anxiety and pain, you are taking action to embrace all the things you've tried to bury and hide over the years. This is how you give breath and space to your being so you can own your light.

CHAPTER THREE

Illumination: Rekindling Your Brightness

Wherever you go, there you are.

—JON KABAT-ZINN, AMERICAN PROFESSOR AND AUTHOR

YOU ARE AMAZING. You've been through so much in your life even if you don't acknowledge or recognize it. You've come so far and moved through so many experiences and stages in your life. You are fascinating and complex, and I can't wait for you to get to know yourself better! Starting in chapter 4, I'll begin referring you to specific practices that will move you in this direction. As you become more intimate with your inner being, you will discover the most interesting person you've ever known. Every day is an adventure when you work on the most important relationship of your life. You will learn to admire your own strength, encourage yourself to be courageous, treat yourself with kindness and compassion, listen to the cues that come to you from your own body, your own intuition, and your own heart, and you will step into the flow of your own life, learn your own rhythm, and have faith in your path to live a life more joyful and peaceful than any you have ever known before.

But how do you do it? How do you meet this person you know has always been inside you, whom you have some general ideas about, but whom you may never have really committed to knowing as well as you could? In this chapter, we're going to get you burning bright by connecting you back to yourself.

~~~~

SURRENDERING TO YOURSELF

The word *surrender* might sound weak or passive to you, but surrender is the path to brightness. Surrender is the key to serenity. It takes great strength and courage because it means giving up the thing that most of us put an extreme value on: control. To surrender means giving up control of what you have no control over and letting things be what they're going to be. To surrender is to accept what is and to change only what you can.

That doesn't mean you ever give up or stop showing up. It's the opposite, in fact. Surrender means you trust that you can release control and open up to the infinite possibilities of the moment in front of you. When you surrender, you will see that you couldn't possibly be anything other than what you are right now. When you surrender, everything gets so much easier! Have faith that there are reasons for what is happening, even if you can't see them. Know that you are here to create good in the world, even if you don't know how you're going to do it yet. Believe that everything is going to be the way it is meant to be, for your highest good and the good of all beings.

When you surrender control, you can see the world as it really is—and that's something you can work with. When you're fooling yourself about reality, all your attempts at manipulating it will be for nothing because you're manipulating phantoms. But when you surrender to truth, the false nature of your fear becomes obvious. Your imprints become obvious. The stories you've been telling yourself about yourself begin to sound ridiculous. You develop a deep compassion for yourself and all you've been through, a compassion you couldn't feel when you were too busy trying to control everything. You can look back on your life and you can understand why you felt so much pain when you did—it's because you were hurt, physically or emotionally or both. As long as you deny your pain and feelings, you can't feel compassion for yourself for having them. When you surrender to what has happened to you and to how you felt about it, the love you can feel for yourself will flood your heart.

You will also see that the past is the past. For you, it may be time to let that be. Surrender what was and stop hanging on to it. Let it go. Learn from it. Release it. Untie yourself from it. Forgive yourself or others. Forgiveness is its own form of personal surrender. You aren't surrendering to whoever hurt you. You are surrendering the pain of that experience. That doesn't mean you forget. Your past is a teacher, but you don't have to take the past with you into the present or into the future. You can leave those imprints behind you, like a wrapper you tossed into the trash can as you went on your way. It's no longer serving you and has no use where you are going.

When students who come to my classes to learn Reiki (an energy-healing practice you will learn more about starting on page 218), and first hear about surrender, I can see them fighting the idea in their own minds. Especially to the ones who have never done yoga or a meditation practice, surrender sounds like being passive, and they don't think they came to me to be passive. They want to learn Reiki and they have a lot of ideas about what they want it to do for them, but the whole idea with Reiki, and all energy work, is surrender. You let go and let whatever is meant to come through come through, for the purpose of balance and harmony. Surrendering to your life in this moment right here and now will lay the groundwork for the surrender necessary to practice Reiki, on yourself or others.

People in recovery from addiction know that the first of the twelve steps of Alcoholics Anonymous (AA) is to admit their powerlessness. This is also a form of surrender. Addiction is a symptom of anxiety. It's an attempt to control pain by covering it up. To surrender is to admit that you can't control pain and that you can't cover it up without repercussions. All you can do if you want the pain to pass is to feel it. Surrender to the feelings. You have them for a reason. They are part of life. Let them rage through you, and then they will move on. They will release their hold on you.

My Reiki master colleague Jen had a profound experience with surrender. After she got married, she and her husband began trying to have a baby. Weeks passed, then months, and then years. All around her, her friends were getting pregnant. Every time someone said something like "Oops, I accidentally got pregnant again," it filled her with pain. At first, she became very controlling of her efforts to get pregnant. She sees that now, looking back. Her root chakra (page 213) was blocked because she didn't trust anything. She didn't know the universe was supporting her and she didn't understand that surrender was something she could even think about. She began to have infertility treatments. She had to admit to doctor after doctor that she wasn't getting pregnant. It was devastating for her. After years of working with doctors, Jen and her husband finally saw a specialist, and, when that happened, she recognized that she had to let go. She had to surrender and trust and have faith in what her life was going to be. She believed that there was a higher intelligence in the universe that had led her to the specialist, and that now she had to let go and let the specialist take over. Most of all, she had to surrender to an outcome she knew she could not control.

Ultimately, Jen and her husband decided that they would do what the specialist suggested. They would try intrauterine insemination (IUI) and then in vitro fertilization (IVF), and if those didn't work, they would stop trying. They would see it as a sign that it wasn't meant to be. They decided they could be okay as a childless couple, that they would survive, and that their marriage would survive. She and her husband both surrendered to her body, to the doctor, and to the universe. With the IUI, Jen got pregnant and she was ecstatic, but it was an ectopic pregnancy and she lost the baby. She was devastated yet again. She had one chance left. That was IVF. The IVF worked, and today her son Wyatt is six years old.

Jen says that if it hadn't worked, she would have had to accept that and she would have found peace with it, but she also believes that when she finally let go of the outcome, she relaxed into the supportive arms of a higher power and her deepest wish was fulfilled.

My friend Katie also had a deep surrender experience after her parents and her husband all died four years ago. She was filled with grief and consumed by fear, especially of the future. She felt like the three people who had given her life its foundation and whom she loved the most (other than her children) had abandoned her, and she couldn't see how her life could ever have any joy in it again. She felt alone, even in a room full of people. Katie tried many things—medication helped her to function and sleep at first, but it didn't address the underlying grief. Therapy was helpful, but more as a tool for helping her children cope and helping her maneuver through the practical aspects of her life alone. But none of these reached her at a spiritual level, which is where the pain was.

I met Katie when she reached out to me after a workshop of mine that she attended. We had done some deep healing work with meditation, Reiki, and crystals, and something inside Katie shifted—something she never knew was in there. She felt a reconnection to her inner being and her faith. She knew she had found something that was going to help restore the joy in her life. By looking deep within herself and feeling what was inside her, Katie was finally able to fully feel her grief and fear, and understand where it had most deeply impacted her. She was able to bring awareness to what had happened to her, and, in doing that, she was able to release its hold on her soul.

To begin surrendering, all you have to do is "effort" less. By that I mean, stop making everything so hard. Stop fighting what is and stop fighting who you are. Stop pushing things away that you know could be good for you and stop clinging to things that you know hurt you. It's easy to surrender the small things. It's hard to surrender the big things, as Jen and Katie experienced. But surrender is the path to serenity.

I often remind myself and the students I'm teaching to stop rushing through life. What do you think is going to happen or not happen if you stop doing all the time and enjoy your life? If, instead of pushing yourself and not sleeping to get that project done for work, what if you rested instead? What if I told you that someone else's urgency is not your urgency?

That doesn't mean you don't take responsibility for the things you've agreed to and committed to, but it does mean that you have a choice and you are the one responsible for what you choose to take on from others. If you don't finish something on time because you are exhausted, it's okay. The truth is, most people are self-focused, and most of the time, they have no interest in what you're doing because they're more focused on what you think of what *they're* doing.

Just let things be—people, circumstances, feelings. Act according to who you are and what you need, and let go of all the rest of it. Observe yourself and your reactions to life, rather than trying to control and shape everything. Observation is a good way to practice surrender. You can exist in the present moment with full awareness, and when you do so with surrender, you will see a whole new world. Colors look brighter. Everything looks sharper, as if it were just coming into focus. You may recognize your gratitude for things you haven't noticed before, like the trees on your daily drive to work, or the water coming out of your morning shower. The beauty and the meaning in these things start to grow exponentially. It's an amazing feeling when you finally stop effort-ing all the time and just start living in the natural flow of your life.

When you exist in the present moment with *inner* awareness, you really *feel* things. You feel when you are deeply exhausted. You feel when you have energy flowing through you and you are ready to take action. You can even feel what foods you need, what movements you need, and what kinds of things you need to say to yourself to make yourself recognize that where you are right now is perfect and purposeful and you are never doing anything the wrong way or at the wrong time. It's all an opportunity to get in sync with your natural rhythms.

When you surrender in your daily life, you'll meet the people who are meant to be on the journey with you, and you won't have to force the connection. You will know how to serve. You will feel the ways in which you belong in the world, rather than fighting to find your place in it. Your intuition will have the space and quiet it needs to become useful. You will begin to see guidance, direction, indicators of rightness, and beautiful synchronicities all around you. And you will see that we are all here with the same sense of human-ness, with the same basic needs, desires, and cravings for a sense of purpose, love, community, and belonging. This will bring greater compassion into your heart.

All this awareness gifts you with information that you can trust because it came to you without you trying to control its content. It came out of all the resources you have to spare when you stop fighting. It came out of surrender.

CHECK-IN TIME:

Let's take a moment so that you can pause and check in with yourself. Take some deep breaths and focus inward. How are you feeling? Don't judge, just notice.

TAKING CARE OF YOU

You probably hear it all the time: "Self-care, self-care, self-care. Put on your own oxygen mask before helping others." This is one of those things that a lot of people say, but very few people actually do with any commitment. Self-care starts with awareness. Without awareness, you are more likely to do what you think you *should* do for yourself, or what other people have told you that you *should* do for yourself, rather than what you really need.

My friend Lea used to think that self-care just meant one thing: exercise. If she didn't go to the gym, she thought she wasn't taking care of herself, even though she exercised so much and so hard that sometimes she felt exhausted and depleted. She might get a massage every few months, too. But over the last few years (and following a few lectures from me!) she has come to see that self-care can mean a lot more than physical care. Sometimes, you just need to give yourself a break. Sometimes you just need to say no to any more obligations. Sometimes you just need to take a day off, or meditate, or hang out with your friends for an afternoon. Sometimes, self-care can mean pushing yourself to go out and get something you really want, or say yes to doing something you might not otherwise do, just to bring more connection and stimulation into your life when you are feeling stagnant and stuck. Self-care can mean meditation or a pedicure, prayer or laughter, a big fresh salad or a scrumptious ice cream sundae. Only you can feel it, by opening yourself to inner awareness.

If you aren't sure, start with some basics. Eat a healthy, balanced meal or try going off sugar and alcohol for a month. Take a break from constant productivity. Even if there are just a couple of moments in the day when you need to lie down on the couch and replenish, do that. Taking care of you means finding a rhythm and cadence for your life. Your inner resources are sacred, so when you use them, use them well, and when they are running low, replenish them. You have rhythms for a reason. You aren't meant to be busy all the time and you aren't meant to rest all the time. There is a balance, and you have a balance that is uniquely yours. It will keep changing over time and in different seasons of your life. Expand your awareness, my love, so you can feel what you need, and then give it to yourself. You are most deserving of this feeling.

~~~~~~

FACING THE STORM

With awareness of the beauty and harmony of life also comes awareness of the experiences and feelings you don't necessarily want to have—grief, pain, fear, doubt, anger. When you first begin trying to feel your feelings, your mind may object. You may find yourself doing almost anything to avoid feeling something that hurts you or makes you feel emotional or uncertain. The mind will even try to distract you from feeling so much that it may mean staying in a destructive thought pattern or a bad situation. You may deny your feelings, or argue with anyone who tries to point them out to you. You may even argue with yourself! This is a protective mechanism, but this is also your chance to break free of those old imprints and programs, so stay with me here.

Experiencing strong feelings is like experiencing a storm. One way is to pretend there isn't a storm happening at all. This may be what you were doing before. You draw the blinds, close the curtains, and put on your noise-canceling headphones. You go about your business, all the while telling yourself that there isn't anything tearing off the roof of your house and knocking over the trees in your yard. You pretend that your street isn't flooding and your neighbors aren't pounding on the door, asking for shelter. You keep telling yourself: "Everything is fine, I'm okay, I'm good. No, really—everything is fine, I'm okay, I'm good." But everything isn't fine. It's okay that everything isn't fine. To feel your feelings is to let yourself *feel* that everything isn't fine. But storms are scary, so even though, deep down, you know there is a storm, you might try as hard as you can not to know it— and that disharmony is what has been creating anxiety, pain, and burnout.

Instead, to break through the fear and feel the storm, embrace the storm. Surrender to the storm. Know its impermanence. Give yourself permission to go on that dark journey. The storm is beautiful, even when it involves change, temporary pain, and the unknown. You can experience this awesomeness if you let it pass over you without trying to tell the storm to stop storming. Rather, you can change and adjust and move as the storm moves. This isn't about letting a storm destroy you and your life, or about being passive. It's about accepting reality for what it is so you can make the changes and adjustments you need to grow and change because of how the storm has changed your inner landscape. If the roof is off your house, look up and see that the roof is off your house. That is the only way you will know that you have to fix it. The journey through feeling always ends in light, eventually. When storms are over, the clouds part and the sun comes out again. This is what life is—a naturally rhythmic, rising-and-falling series of opportunities to stand in wonderment at the gifts and lessons of life's experiences.

This is not a quick-fix process, which is why I never teach "five hacks to happiness" or "change your life in thirty days." You're much bigger and deeper than five hacks or thirty days. What is happening to you when you feel strong feelings and let yourself have transformative experiences is not trivial. You have lived an entire life, filled with millions of feelings and experiences. To believe that you can heal and shift and change everything in one month or even in one year would be to dishonor the incredible and complex journey of your life. Storms and gorgeous days and everything in between are wondrous and amazing, and they are all part of the long winding path from fear, exhaustion, pain, grief, and darkness to burning bright.

Remember that change is your friend, and storms don't last. Every storm is temporary. Every strong feeling is temporary. But denial is not temporary if you choose to cling to it. Strong feelings will always dissipate, just as a storm does. Pretending that you can control the sky or deny the storm can cause incredible pain. You can't cling to a hurricane. You can't hold on to it like a kite on a string.

The hurricane doesn't have anything to do with you. It's just passing through your experience, and you can't decide when it will start or when it will end. You can accept it or deny it, but it won't change what is actually happening. Once you face the storm, you will see that, even if it was terrible, it didn't last forever. In every moment, at every perceived crisis, you can always choose to fight and resist it, to deny it, to regret it, to fear it, or to be angry about it . . . or you can choose to accept it with love and a willingness to evolve and grow and learn from the challenge, seeing where it takes you. I want you to give yourself permission to feel what you feel, but also permission to understand that what you're feeling doesn't mean anything about you, or about where you're going or who you will be or all the wonderful things that you will do in life.

You won't always be happy. You won't enjoy losing your job or a relationship or whatever it is. You probably don't want to stand in the middle of a hurricane. But life is not about constant, undisturbed happiness, and the hurricane is full of gifts. When I left my job in the US Senate at the lowest point in my life, it turned out to be the greatest move I ever made. It changed my life, and now I love where I am, who I am, and what I do. I never would have found this path if I hadn't come to the place where I still live today, where everything was different from any place I'd ever been before.

When I was in my twenties, I had no idea that it would ever be enough for me to just show up in my life as myself. I would make up these scenarios about all the things I had to do all the time to be a better person. I would think, *If I go to somebody's house for a dinner party, I need to make sure I offer to clean the dishes*, or *I'll take the daughter outside to play on the playground so her mom isn't stressed out*, even though what I really wanted was to stay and enjoy the party and the people. I didn't know how to feel safe just being me because I was too busy trying to control some idea of who I thought I should be.

So you lost your job? Congratulations. So your relationship is over? Congratulations. So you got kicked out of school, or failed the bar exam, or you stopped speaking to your parents? Congratulations. Now you know something you didn't know before about yourself. If the stressful thing that happens to you brings up all your fears, congratulations. Now you have the opportunity to surrender to the feelings of fear so they can pass through you and move on. The minute that you focus your energy inward and choose to do the work on yourself and get curious about your feelings, you change. You shift. And you get closer to who you really are. That's when things start happening with ease and grace, when abundance comes to you, when you find love, and health, and the physical, mental, and emotional resources you need. When you effort less, you can receive more.

When you can ride the ups and downs of your life's waves with a sense of ease and trust in the rightness of your journey, you will learn to inhabit your entire body, your thoughts, your pain, and your discomfort, as well as your joy, your sense of rightness and worthiness, and the knowledge that you matter. There is an appropriate quote often attributed to Johann Wolfgang von Goethe: "As soon as you trust yourself, you will know how to live." That, my dear, is at the heart of surrender.

VIBE

As you practice feeling your feelings, sometimes you might begin to feel overwhelmed or afraid. When that happens, just VIBE with it. Ask yourself these four questions and you can calm your mind and be empowered to keep feeling:

V: Am I playing the victim right now?
When you feel afraid, you may begin to think that you are the victim of your fear or of whatever has caused the fear. Instead, choose to be the hero of your situation. Remember this Nelson Mandela quote: "Courage is not the absence of fear, but the triumph over it."

I: What is my intuition telling me about this situation?
Get quiet and calm and go inside. As the feelings wash over you, ask your internal wisdom what's really going on. Strong feelings can cloud your judgment of the situation, but your intuition knows what's really going on. Remember this Madeleine L'Engle quote: "Don't try to comprehend with your mind. Our minds are very limited. Use your intuition."

B: Who do I want to be in this situation?
Don't worry about who you think you are or how well you are handling the situation in the middle of an intense feeling. Your imprints can mislead you about that. Instead, look to who you would *want to be* as you feel this feeling, and see the situation through that lens.

E: What would empower me right now in this situation?
Think of one thing you can do right now that will make you feel strong and powerful. If you are feeling anxiety, try practicing EFT (page 167) or going for a walk. If you are feeling fear, try stepping outside and looking at the sky, or journaling. If you are feeling grief, stop holding back the tears and let yourself cry it out, or take long, deep breaths until the feeling starts to pass through you. The only thing that won't empower you is muffling the feeling back down again. Remember that it will only come back up later, so you might as well get it all out right now.

FINDING YOUR NATURAL RHYTHM

Nature is rhythmic—the ebb and flow of ocean waves, the chirping of birds, the beat of rain, the music of a flowing river, the random rhythms of the wind, and the way the earth spins so that, in our perception, the sun and moon rise and set in a slow dance of light and darkness across the planet. You have a rhythm, too, and when you stop doing and start feeling, you will feel that rhythm. Your rhythm is part of who you are, and it is unique to you. You don't control it. You aren't the conductor of your rhythm. You are the instrument that produces the rhythm. Listen, and you will hear it and feel it from within.

Your rhythm has ups and it has downs. That means, at some points in your life, you will feel happy, joyful, euphoric, and at other times you will feel low and sad. Sometimes you will feel pain and experience difficulty. This is how life works and how nature works. We've all experienced this.

When I go out and speak to a crowd or lead a retreat, I am on a high of energy and connection, but when I come home, I almost always experience a crash. It can feel like a letdown if I don't remind myself that this is part of the natural rhythm. A wave rises up, peaks, then falls into a trough. This is how energy works.

It's the same for a singer who goes on tour and has the high of a great show and then crashes between shows. It's the same for a woman who is pregnant. The energy builds and builds and peaks at the birth, but then sometimes there's a crash, which can result in things like postpartum depression. You might have an amazing vacation or go to an awesome party or meet someone new and feel swept away by romance, but those feelings don't last. After the vacation, after the party, after the first few months of a new relationship, you will probably experience the trough of the wave. You might feel sad or disappointed or just need more rest than usual. This also happens to a lot of people after the holiday season, after a wedding, or on their birthdays. They build up to a peak and then they crash.

The peak of the wave isn't always something fun or beautiful. Sometimes it is a tragedy. On a retreat I was recently leading, there was a girl whose father had suddenly passed away just three months before. They had worked together every day, and she felt that he was her one ally in her family. She was shocked that he had died, and was still feeling a lot of pain and sadness, but she felt that she should be over it by that time and back to living her regular life. This idea of the waves helped her—I explained that the feeling of the wave crashing down, and the sadness that she felt, was natural, and part of the rhythm of her life. It was okay to grieve, and she could give herself permission to continue grieving for as long as she needed to. She was in the trough beneath the wave, but eventually the energy would come back up. And, of course, she was still grieving; how could the loss of her father be resolved in three months? Still, the pain was difficult for her, so I asked her if she could think about a shift: What if, instead of feeling his absence, she could fill herself up with his love and the part of him that was inside her every day? This way, she could grieve his physical absence, but still feel him with her. This can help regulate the energy, bringing it gradually back up again, in its natural time.

It's all worthy of awareness. You can't allow the wave but deny the trough, or submit to the sea when it is calm but turn away when the waves get bigger. The sea is always there, whether you look at it or not, so you might as well look at it. This is all as it should be. The rhythm is within you at every moment, big and small. You have large waves and tiny ripples but they are all a rhythm. You can begin to tune in to your own rhythm just by listening to the rhythm of your breath. Sit quietly for a few minutes. Feel your breath moving in and out of your body. See if you can feel or sense the beat of your heart, the throb of your pulse, the flow of your blood. It's all the rhythm.

Your internal rhythm is your oasis. It is entirely yours. As you become more awake to the present moment of your life, you will be able to observe what other people do and how they live in or out of their own rhythms. This is not to judge them or their journey, but rather to see a mirror. Some of them will seem lost. Others will seem brilliant and you may be inspired by them. Who was the last person you noticed or met who seemed to have a light on inside them? Maybe you couldn't explain it or recognize why that person seemed so bright, but you felt it. That is someone who is in their natural rhythm. Life is a miracle, and each being is playing a part in the infinite cycle of being. When you let your life flow in its natural rhythm, receiving and allowing instead of pushing and blocking and struggling, you will enter a state of harmony and feel your own infinite depths.

~~~~~

NOT-DOING

Sitting quietly and listening to the rhythm of your breath is a form of meditation. Many of my students think meditation is hard, especially when they are caught in the cycle of constant doing. Meditation is about sitting and being, rather than moving and doing. You might think it would be easy to stop doing, but it's not. Just sit down and try it. Try sitting for ten minutes without doing anything. No looking at your phone or the TV or a book. No talking to anyone. No planning what you are going to do next. This can drive people crazy because we live in a culture that glorifies doing-ness.

When you first try to not-do, you will probably feel a constant sense of wanting to exit the present moment. You will suddenly feel the urgency to *do something* or *be somewhere else* or *get something done*, because it's hard to just sit and feel. But inside that not-doing is a sense of presence, peace, clarity, and self-love unlike anything you can get from outside yourself. You won't find it if you never stop doing.

You have an unexplored universe inside you, but you can't see it if you are only looking outside you.

How do you get to this inner universe? You can't do something to find it. No one else can show it to you or give it to you. You only need to stop doing to experience how incredible, full, inspiring, easy, energizing, and nourishing not-doing is for your soul. This is the space where you can discover yourself and your true nature. This is how you know what you need in your life, and this is where you can explore to determine how to live on the outside in accordance with who you are on the inside. To not-do is to look within yourself rather than outside yourself.

You may not be able to stay there for long at first, but if you step inside yourself regularly, you will find that you can stay there longer each time. You don't have to run from this. It's the most wonderful place in the world to be. Eventually, this delicious not-doing-ness will be with you even when you are doing. You can take little breaks to enjoy it. Take just ten minutes (or a weekend) to stop looking at your phone, stop planning, stop responding, stop knowing what you're going to have for dinner, stop trying to solve a problem . . . stop trying to *create* a problem or a need or anything you have to ask of yourself. Just be, and see what happens. The world is always in motion and something will happen. Go with it and see where it takes you.

This is a basic state of being that you will use when you start practicing Reiki and other healing techniques later on. You can channel universal healing energy through you if your mind is not constantly getting in the way. Later in this book, I'll show you how to do many of these practices, to keep clearing the way for the energy you need to live in a state of peace and flow, but, for now, just practice this not-doing and see where you can apply it in your life each day, even if it's just for a few moments at first.

Be ready for that resistance, that made-up chaos that your imprints generate when you begin to shift—you may feel a resistance to putting down your phone, resistance to ease, resistance to quiet and space, resistance to joy in your daily life. Just stop resisting and all the feelings will happen and then pass. Just stop effort-ing, again and again. This is a powerful practice that doesn't even feel like a practice, because it's the opposite of a practice. It's the absence of a practice and the presence of being.

When I explain this state to my students, sometimes they ask me how, if they aren't doing anything, they can ever accomplish anything. Not-doing is a basic practice that can help you to begin shifting internally, according to what is authentic and right for you, but it doesn't mean you literally won't do anything ever again. It means that you give yourself the space and awareness to recognize what you really *want* to do, as opposed to what you think you *should* do. The result is that you begin to live your life according to your authentic needs and desires, rather than the demands of the external world.

Let's say that your friend is having a big birthday dinner, and even though you love your friend, you feel exhausted. When you go inside yourself, you recognize that you just don't want to go to that big birthday dinner. You could force yourself to go, or you could tell your friend that you can't make it, even though the only reason you can't make it is because you are feeling exhausted. What you really want to do is take a bath and read a good book or watch your favorite TV show. You might fear that your friend will be upset or disappointed, but if you force yourself to go to the party, you could end up feeling sick the next day.

To not-do the party means to do something that feels more in line with what you need in the moment, and that is okay. Often, it leads to something better than what you decided not to do. Maybe you tell your friend you love them so much and are sorry to miss out on the special night, but that you are just depleted and need a night in. Then, maybe a few days later, the two of you end up having a one-on-one dinner together that becomes the most beautiful, magical, and wonderful night as friends that you have ever had together, at a level much more in sync with who you are and what you need and the nature of your particular friendship with this person. Your anxiety and fear might make you believe that you don't have a choice but to go to the party, but your heart and your higher self know there could be a more incredible experience waiting for just the two of you if you choose to not-do.

When you only do what feels right for your natural rhythm, doing stops causing anxiety. You can have all the experiences you want to have while letting resistance and control and struggle go. What you are not-doing is fighting. What you *are* doing is living, feeling, and focusing on actions in harmony with your true nature. What you focus on grows, and you will get more of it, whatever it is, so focus on the things you want. Sometimes that means focusing on the big feelings inside so that you can give them permission to transmute, shift, and heal. Once you get clear, you can use this power of intention to move in the direction of a more authentic life for yourself, filled with all the things you desire.

THE PUSH AND PULL OF DESIRE

Is it okay to want things? Isn't it selfish? Desire can be confusing. People often feel greedy when they focus on their desires, but superficial desires are usually just symbols of something deeper that your soul craves, and what your soul craves is never greedy.

Let's say you think you want more money. What you really want may be freedom to spend your time following your passions rather than just earning a living, or abundance in all aspects of your life, or to ease your worry about providing for your family. If you think you want to get married, what you really want may be deep human connection, or support, or relief from loneliness. If you think you want a better career, what you really want may be the fulfillment that comes from doing work that has meaning for you, or relief from a stressful situation or difficult people. If you think you want to change some aspect of your physical body, what you really want may be to love yourself unconditionally.

One of my clients and dear friends, Stacie, went through this with me. For years, she drove an old car with 200,000 miles on it. It worked, but it wasn't reliable. This was all Stacie could afford when she was struggling in her career, but after working together to break through some creative blocks and channel her energy to be more in line with her gifts of acting and singing, she had doubled her income. But she was still driving that old car.

The car she truly desired was a white Lexus SUV with tan seats, but she felt guilty about buying that. She told me, "Who am I to drive a luxury car? I'm not super-wealthy." So she kept putting it off. I could feel that this wasn't aligned for her and I kept telling her, "Stacie, listen to that whisper before it becomes a scream," but she didn't. She felt that she didn't deserve the car, and that her desire was too frivolous or vapid.

One day, Stacie walked out her front door to go to work, and her car was gone. She was sure it had been stolen. She called the police to report the crime, only to discover that the car had been towed because she had never changed her Nevada license plates and registration over to California. It was going to cost her $800 to get her car back. She called me and said, "I can't afford this! Why did this happen to me?!"

"Oh my, girl," I said, "you didn't listen to the whisper. You let it become a scream. Will you listen now?" Within a week, Stacie sold her old car and leased a new Lexus. It has never once been the financial burden she feared it would be. This new car makes her feel safe, confident, and, most of all, worthy. *That* is what the car was really about. Even more important, Stacie learned to listen to that inner voice telling her that she was worthy of the car she needed. She now likes to say that this whole lesson was much bigger than any car—that it has helped her step into who she is today.

You don't always have to recognize the inner truths behind your desires to let go of guilt. Just have faith and trust that there are many layers behind the money, the marriage, the career, the health, or even the new Lexus you desire, and that all those layers are trying to shift you into harmony with who you really are, beyond your fear, beyond your imprints, beyond your doubts about your own worthiness, all the way down to the depths of your soul—that part of you that is filled with light and knowing and purposeful intention.

Contrary to what your fear might tell you, moving toward your desires doesn't require struggle or striving. As Stacie learned, what is more difficult is not listening to them, because that is when you are in disharmony, and things will just get harder. Instead, see yourself as already living your desired reality with ease and grace. If it helps you, you could reframe your desire into a more holistic framework: abundance instead of wealth, connection instead of marriage, fulfillment instead of success, energy instead of weight loss, or whatever it is for you. Feel that word in your heart. Let it move outward from your heart through your veins and into every cell, every bone, tendon, organ, muscle, and fiber in your body. See yourself as if that word were your reality. It's not a race. It's not effort. It's just an intention you are putting out there. And it starts with your belief that you are worthy of receiving it.

In the practice of energy healing that is Reiki, there is something called the Reiki precepts, which I'll tell you more about in chapter 7, but basically, these are phrases you tell yourself for guidance in living a well-balanced and healthy life. They begin with "Just for today," such as "Just for today, I will not anger," and "Just for today, I will not worry."

A few years ago, when I was struggling with big changes in my life and nothing felt easy, I felt as if I didn't have any grace, so I decided to make my own precept. Every morning, I said to myself, "Just for today, I am ease and grace." I vowed to say it daily even if I didn't feel that it was having any effect. At first it seemed a little far-fetched, but I kept at it until it became a habit. I didn't even think about what might happen if it would work. I just kept saying it.

One day, about two years later, I was doing my daily practice, and I said, "Just for today, I am ease and grace," and then I stopped and smiled and almost laughed. I realized suddenly that everything in my life *did* feel easy. My life *did* feel graceful. I was there, finally, and I hadn't even realized how the transformation happened. But it did happen. It took me some time to get there, but I got there. Just speaking the words, setting the intention, and being consistent worked.

What do you want to be, just for today, without expectations or attachments to the outcome you have planned in your head? Do you want to be strong, soft, calm, passionate, peaceful, open, energized, engaged? Tell yourself in your mind: "Just for today, I am . . ." Add your just-for-today word, and feel it. See it. Infuse it into your mind. Send it out into the world. Then—and this is the most important part—let it go, with no attachment to the outcome. Then do it all again tomorrow.

No attachment to the outcome means you won't be waiting around all day for that check to arrive in the mail, or to bump into your soul mate, or for your family to start suddenly getting along, or for that perfect job opportunity or that perfect new house or that perfect dream vacation to just suddenly become available. Instead, trust that everything is happening the way it is intended to, and in its own time. Where you are now is where you are meant to be, and where you will be tomorrow will also be right. When it's time for those good things to come to you, they will come to you, and if they don't come to you, there is a reason and a lesson in that, too. Just keep your mind on what you want for your life, believe in your ability to become this you, and go with your life's flow to get you there. The rest will take care of itself.

Of course, it's not quite as simple as it sounds. It's not just pure magic. Focus and intention are complex. It may feel as if you are only thinking about what you want and not doing anything about it, but that focus and that intention actually change how you exist in the world, and how others around you exist, too. Think about this: Let's say you're struggling to make enough money and you worry about money all the time. You have anxiety about making enough, having enough, meeting your obligations. This anxiety and focus on lack of financial resources can have a subtle effect on everything around you, including you. It could cause you to make multiple, almost imperceptibly small money decisions that make your situation worse. Your anxiety about money may cause you to miss subtle opportunities that could pay off later. It could influence how you appear to other people, which could cause you to lose jobs or get paid less because you are projecting the energy of deficiency and desperation. You may be attracting deficiency to you in ways you don't even realize, or pushing away abundance without knowing it.

But if your focus is on abundance, and if you say to yourself, "Just for today, I allow myself to receive radiant abundance in every way," and you really let your mind live in that space, you will project a completely different quality of energy that can tune you in to opportunities, attract people who might offer help, and change the way people respond to you in ways that could pay off big later.

Think about Stacie and her car. There was a reason that she never changed her registration from the old Nevada plates. The car represented her old life, which she was still hanging on to, but even without realizing it, she was already loosening her grip on that past life. She knew, at least at some level, that when you move to a new state, you have to change your registration. Not doing that was a way of letting the car go—her feelings about the car subtly influenced what she did with that car, which influenced what happened to that car, and then, there it went, towed away to send her the most obvious message: It's time for something new.

You can choose fear-based living, or you can choose love-based living, where you allow things to come in and out with a sense of ease and faith that all is right on time. That doesn't mean you're going to quit working or paying your bills or having relationships. You are meant to experience life with all your energy and allow the light moving inside you to be active, connected, and engaged with the world. To effort less means to live more openly, with a full willingness to experience this life you've been gifted. Instead of resisting work, you can do your work with love, ease, and joy. Instead of avoiding conflicts in relationships, you can engage with other people with a sense of calm and openness to your feelings, letting the conflicts happen and pass so nothing stays buried. Instead of resisting your bills, you can pay them peacefully to the best of your ability.

I noticed recently that whenever I wrote checks out for my business, I was gripping my pen and writing so hard that my back would tense up. Huh? Why would I do that? I never noticed it before, but when I sat with it for a few minutes, I realized that I've never liked writing checks or paying out money, even though I deeply appreciate and respect the people I work with and it's a beautiful and necessary exchange. I realized that writing out checks brought up an old imprint of fear around money. My parents used to talk about money a lot and my dad would balance his checkbook every single weekend, and sometimes every day. He would always hesitate or make comments when he wrote a check, sometimes for my dance recital costumes. Instead of seeing the beauty and joy in having money in my account to pay people, I was letting this old fear program run me and I didn't even know it until I allowed myself to become aware of it and take responsibility to change it.

CHECK-IN TIME:

Let's take a moment so that you can pause and check in with
yourself. Take some deep breaths and focus inward. How are
you feeling? Don't judge, just notice.

COMPARING YOURSELF TO YOURSELF

Do you believe that who you were at some point in the past or who you could be sometime in the future is better than who you are right now? It's not true. If you believe that today, when you don't want to get off the couch, you are not as good as you were yesterday, when you had energy, then you are living according to external beliefs about yourself. Instead, acting from internal rather than external cues will help you feel your own nature in every moment as you constantly change and as your needs shift. Maybe, today, it's more important for you to rest than to exercise, but an old program may tell you that you are *always* a better person when you exercise than you are when you don't exercise, or that the you who is *doing* is always better than the you who is resting. If you say unkind things to yourself whenever you aren't acting according to your own ideas about worthiness (ideas that come from imprints), you are missing the chance to bring awareness to who you are right now in this moment.

The truth is that where you were at any other moment in your fascinating and ever-changing life isn't relevant to who you are in this moment. There is no "bad" you and "good" you. There is only you. The you of yesterday is no better or worse than the you of tomorrow, no matter what you are doing now and what you did then. The you who was ten pounds lighter or was in the flow at work is no better than the you who is sad or "not fit" or nervous or self-doubting. The you who received lots of "comments" and "likes" on social media is no better than the you who scrolled on social media for two hours, feeling bad about yourself as you looked at other people's "amazing" lives and stories. Whether you feel good or bad, whether you are moving or sleeping, arguing with a friend/partner/child or hugging them, eating a doughnut or eating a salad, it's just you. Happy, healthy you is no better or worse than you going through a rough patch. And this is *always true*.

This doesn't mean you can't move in directions you prefer or become the person you dream of becoming. You can do anything you want to do, to feel better or improve your circumstances. You can look at those times when you were doing well and examine what was happening then. You can move and create change now to get toward that state again, just as the ocean rises up into waves, then sinks into troughs, then rises up again. Just remember that each day and each week and each year and each moment will be different. That's the beauty of change and surrender—letting go of what was in order to embrace ups and downs and natural rhythms of what is, and allowing this to become part of your beautiful human journey. If you embrace all parts of yourself and acknowledge what you need in this moment, then you will know who you are—not then, not before, but right now.

ACCESSING INTUITION

Intuition is your wise inner guide that points you in the right direction, according to what you need and desire. Intuition tells you when to act and when to rest, when to say yes and when to say no. Your intuition can advise you in any situation, but people often don't listen to it, or trust it, or they think they need the intuition of others to guide them. Your intuition is a quiet voice, so you may have to get quiet in order to hear it, but you have your own intuition, I promise you. Intuition comes from deep within you, from that inner authentic self that isn't governed by your imprints or your fear. While the intuition of others, such as teachers and mentors, can sometimes help you see more deeply into your own intuition, you are never without your inner guide.

Intuition works best when the mind and the heart are synchronized. The mind is like the mail carrier—it receives the mail, or the information. The heart is what reads the letters and digests the words to determine what you should do with the information. This can happen very quickly. Your mind might take in the information: "That bus is going really fast toward this crosswalk!" Your heart immediately reads this information and sends out a warning: "It's not safe to step into the street!" Even before you consciously notice the speeding bus, this process may give you a feeling that you should wait on the curb for just a little longer than you might have. Listen to your intuition because it knows more than your conscious mind.

If the mind were acting alone, it might spiral down a rabbit hole about something that has nothing to do with where you are right now, and you might never notice that speeding bus coming down the street, or your mind might see the bus and panic and go into control-and-fear mode, having you believe you are going to get hit by the bus no matter what you do, even if you are still standing safely on the sidewalk. The mind working alone to control your environment gets in the way of intuition, but when the mind and intuition work together, you will be able to act with more clarity.

Many people have told me stories about how their intuition guided them in the most mysterious ways. Back when she was eighteen, Jess, a colleague of mine, was an exchange student in France. Her host family thought it would be fun to take her on a ride in a high-speed go-kart. She immediately had the feeling that she shouldn't do it. She literally heard a voice in her head saying, "Don't do it. Don't do it." Jess told her host family no, but the family kept urging her to do it, telling her how much fun she would have, until she finally gave in.

The ride was terrifying. The go-kart driver sped up to 55 miles per hour, and just before he was about to hit a tire wall, he swerved suddenly. Jess was thrown out of the go-kart, tore every tendon in her ankle, and had to go to the hospital. She told me that was the day she learned that she should listen to her intuition, and whenever she questions her inner voice, she reminds herself about that terrible go-kart accident. Jess's intuition tends to come through as an actual inner voice, but yours may come through as a feeling, a sound, a thought, a vision, or a mood. There are so many ways we each uniquely experience our own intuition. No matter how close or how far you feel from yours, it's there and it's always ready to work with you.

Another very close friend of mine, Karen, has a special intuition around people. Many times, she has thought of someone she hadn't thought about for a long time, and then that person will call or text her soon after. She can feel the energy of people passing on the street, and when she hugs someone, sometimes she can feel that she would not want to get to know that person any better, or that they have a deep warmth that makes her want to get to know them. Karen's intuition tends to come through as a palpable sensation of energy quality.

Your intuition can be a powerful ally in your life. It may come through as a voice or a feeling or a sense of knowing. You may see signs or hear songs or notice numbers that your intuition calls to your attention for a reason. Your intuition can tell you what your body needs, what thoughts to follow, and what connections and people are good or bad for you. Should you take that job? Accept that proposal? Move to that city? Explore that new relationship? Your mind acting alone might tell you, "Argue with that obnoxious person!" Your intuition might tell you, "Let it go." Your mind alone might tell you, "You can't take a dance class. You're too clumsy." Your intuition might say, "Why not give it a try? It might really bring you joy." Your intuition will often tell you to act with intention, while the mind alone is more likely to tell you to react. When you are faced with a decision, your intuition knows the answers, which means you know the answer, even if you think at first that you don't.

It's easy to start listening to your intuition. All you have to do is stop *doing* for a minute and listen. Sit quietly and ask yourself any question: *Do I want to try this? Do I want to say no to this? What is the right path right now?* Be as specific as you can with your question, then let the answer rise up from deep inside. If you are listening, you will hear it. It might not come right away, but as soon as you ask, your intuition will begin working on the energy and an answer will come eventually.

You don't have to be sitting and meditating to do this. You can access your intuition at any time. When you wake up in the morning, you can ask yourself: *What do I need today to feel healthy, or calm, or directed, or connected?* Maybe you just need to step outside into the sunshine for fifteen minutes before you go to work. Maybe you need to have a cup of chamomile tea and relax, or write in your journal for a few minutes, or take a bath. Let your intuition guide you—it can help you to take care of yourself in the ways you need the most, so you can live with more balance, well-being, confidence, and trust.

The more you listen to your intuition, the more attuned you will become to its messages. Your intuition will also call your attention to the signs around you. Beautiful synchronicities that are a communication between you and the universe can be glorious or they may seem trivial at first. Maybe you drop your phone in the bathtub. You can flip out and have a moment of anger and anxiety, or you can say, *Wow, that is clearly a message that I am not in the present moment and I need to detach from technology for a while.* If you have a craving for your favorite cookies and the coffee shop is out of them, you can be annoyed, or you can say, *Hmm, I guess I'm not meant to have a cookie today. Sugar is probably not what my body needs right now.* Maybe you are late to class, and you are irritated at yourself for not waking up sooner, but, on the way, you meet someone who becomes an important person in your life, or you avoid an accident on the freeway that would have made you late anyway. Have faith that you are always on time. You are always where you are for a reason.

Some common ways intuition strikes is if you keep hearing a name pop up in random places, or you keep seeing a number everywhere. Perhaps you keep seeing or hearing about a certain type of teacher training or a retreat or a class, and you've had an interest in this or been curious about it for a while. Suddenly, within a week, you see or hear about it from others more than three times. That's your intuition, telling you that it's time. If you are driving and following your GPS, but you suddenly get the feeling that you should go a different way, try it. See what happens. There may be some unexpected joy in that direction, or you may end up avoiding something unpleasant or inconvenient. If you have a dream about someone, tune in to your intuition to see if you are feeling that you should give them a call. You never know how your intuition will communicate to you, but it always communicates in the service of your highest good or the good of others. Just be open to the messages, and you will see that guidance is everywhere.

When I get an intuition, I feel it like a "ping." Sometimes it happens for me and sometimes it happens for someone I am working with. My friend Stacie—the one who wanted the white Lexus—was getting ready for a show after not having performed as a singer for a year. She was having a terrible day. She was nervous, she left her credit card somewhere, she was forgetting the words to the songs that she herself had written—but I had no idea any of this was happening. Suddenly I got a "ping" about Stacie, so I called her. She was at a stoplight in traffic, shaking with anxiety. She said, "How did you know to call me right now?" And then she burst into tears. I did some tapping with her (see page 167) right there on the phone while she sat in standstill traffic at an intersection. Stacie followed my instructions and began tapping on herself. She said it was one of the most connected moments she's ever had, and she never once questioned the magic of it. After that, the rest of the day, and the show, fell perfectly into place.

CHECK-IN TIME:

Let's take a moment so that you can pause and check in with
yourself. Take some deep breaths and focus inward. How are
you feeling? Don't judge, just notice.

INTUITION MODES

There are four main types of intuition. I'm not talking about psychic powers or anything external or unnatural here—these are just names for different modes of inner guidance. Keep an open mind if you can, and just consider whether you think you might relate best to one or two of these forms of intuition. Most of us have a little bit of all of them:

1. Clairsentience: This means "clear feeling." It is the kind of intuition that opens you to sensing the emotions and feelings of other people. You may even have a visceral experience, like a stomachache or a pain in your knee, but it's not really your pain. It's someone else's pain that you are intuiting.

2. Clairvoyance: This one is often misunderstood because there is a Hollywood movie idea of the clairvoyant psychic who tells the future. In reality, *clairvoyance* means "clear seeing," and it is the kind of intuition that manifests as images, like quick snapshots or daydreams, or noticing particular words, signs, or images on billboards or license plates, in books, or just out there in the world. You may see a particular number or series of numbers over and over—this happens to me a lot, so I began to explore numerology to see if I could make more sense of the messages. When you are a visually oriented person, you probably have a clairvoyant intuition.

3. Claircognizance: This means "clear thinking," and it occurs as a deep knowing. Sometimes, you just know something, but you aren't sure how. This knowing can manifest as thoughts that rise up in your mind, or just a sense that you should contact someone or do something or not-do something. Maybe you think of someone right before the phone rings and it's that person calling. This can be easy to miss because we all have so many thoughts every day, but claircognizant intuitions will be slightly louder, more insistent, or have a different energy or feel to them in your mind. If you pay attention, you'll catch them.

4. Clairaudience: When you hear messages, that's clairaudience, which means "clear hearing." You might be the person who hears songs on the radio that seem to answer a question or send a message, or you might find yourself actually singing a song you hadn't thought of in a long time. I have a friend who has this—every time she has some kind of conflict, she realizes that she is humming a song. When she thinks about the lyrics to the song in her mind, it often contains a message, an answer, or a form of guidance. Others might hear a voice and think they are imagining it, but it might be an important message about something you need to do or not-do. Sometimes, clairaudience can happen when you are half asleep or just waking up. You might hear a voice say a word. Sleep scientists call these occurrences sleep hallucinations, but they may contain information for you.

Sometimes it can be hard to figure out if an incoming message is just your mind running an old program or imprint, or if it's really your intuition. Here are some clues: Imprint thinking resists change and reverts back to old patterns and fears, which can keep you in old cycles of behavior or thinking that no longer serve your highest good or help you to grow. Imprint thinking doesn't want to forgive or let go, but, rather, desires to hold on to the past or to concrete beliefs and to keep you stuck, as opposed to forgiving, releasing, accepting, and changing for your highest good. Intuition, on the other hand, allows openness, flow, and change. For example, if you are sitting on the couch thinking, "I really should get up and go for a walk right now," but then you think, "No, no, I feel like I really just want to lie on the couch," and then you think, "No, stop being lazy and get up! You need some exercise!" and then you think, "No, I really think I need to rest," who is who in this internal struggle that could go on and on? Is your mind resisting exercise because of an imprint, or is your intuition telling you that you need rest right now?

To figure it out, get quiet, go inside yourself, and ask yourself: *What am I meant to do right now?* Then let go of any expectation and let your intuition guide you. Sometimes I jot down what I feel when I'm resisting something. I might write: "I'm resisting exercise. Is that right for me?" Don't struggle with the answer. Instead, look for signs. What information is coming in, and how does your heart feel about it?

One clue is which voice is criticizing you and which voice is encouraging you. Imprints criticize and intuition is filled with self-love. But maybe it's not so simple, so be present and observe: Do you notice how beautiful the weather is, and do you suddenly feel called to get out there? Or do you notice that your knee is throbbing and you suddenly feel that it is right to rest after all? If you still don't know, maybe the answer is just to sit and meditate for ten minutes, then see how you feel. If deep down you feel that ping saying you need to move and it is for your highest good, lean into that. If instead you go inward and see that you're feeling depleted and frail inside, lean into that intuition that you need to rest, even if your mind tries to guilt you into more "doing." Tune in to whatever nourishes your body and soul.

When you don't know what to do, you don't need to know what to do. Just wait and don't *do* until you feel guided. Whether or not you exercise on this particular day does not make you or your value in this world any more or less. When you finally quiet the voice of your fear by sitting in stillness and listening, you will be able to hear the voice of your intuition, and know what you need for you. No rush. No pressure. No effort. Just patience and feeling.

It's the same thing if you've been working all day and you know you would benefit from meditating, but you feel as if you *should* keep pushing. Or maybe you've watched three episodes of your favorite reality TV or Netflix show, but you *feel* that your brain is mush and you would be better off turning off the TV, taking a bath, meditating, or making a healthy dinner for yourself and turning some music on instead. Maybe you think you *should* work until midnight, but you *feel* that you *need* to clean up your space and then wind down for sleep. Remember to banish *should* from your vocabulary and focus on *feel*, *want*, *need*, *desire*. Even changing the wording can make you feel better about a plan you have—such as "I should go to this event" as opposed to "I feel led to go to this event" or "I have a plan to go to this event tonight" or even "I'm excited to go to this event." Or "I really don't want to go to this event tonight. Maybe it's not so important for me to go."

The more you take the time and give yourself the space to feel the difference between your imprints and your intuition, the more obvious the difference will become. Just remember that imprints come from external experiences and intuition comes from an openness to your innate inner compass. Your intuition is the gateway to experiencing life's beautiful and effortless flow, and it will gracefully align you to the magic of the present moment.

∿∿∿

GIVING TO YOURSELF

Rekindling your brightness is an act of self-love. It requires nurturing and nourishing yourself, giving yourself space, taking off the pressure. It requires consistency—not the kind of consistency where you punish yourself or blame yourself if you forget or fall off the wagon, but the kind where you just keep coming back with love. This intentional self-love and softening can feel selfish in a busy world, obsessed with productivity, but it's the least selfish thing you can do, because when you burn bright, you will be a beacon for others. When you are filled with the energy of love, harmony, and natural flow, you will be able to reach out and help others from a place of fullness and wholeness. If you are confused, anxious, sad, overextended, and overwhelmed, you won't be able to do much for anyone else, let alone yourself.

Sometimes I find it helpful to remind myself that it is my sacred quest as a human being on this earth to burn bright because that is how to light up the world—and until I take care of myself and nurture and nourish myself, I can't burn bright. So what have you given yourself lately? When I ask my clients, "Why haven't you done more for yourself?," they usually give me at least one of these five excuses:

1. *"I don't have time."*

2. *"I don't know how."*

3. *"I have too many other people who rely on me so I can't be first on my list." (Or "I would feel selfish.")*

4. *"I have too much pain in my physical body to focus on anything else."*

5. *"I can't afford it."*

The second two sections of this book are devoted to the tools, techniques, and rituals you can use to give back to yourself and fill yourself with enormous, bright, infinite light, and you can do almost all of them despite any of these excuses. Some of the techniques take very little time. None require any special knowledge beyond what I give you. They won't take you away from your obligations—you can still live your life while practicing them. All of them help to address and heal physical, mental, and/or spiritual pain, and hardly any of them cost anything. No more excuses! Every time you gift well-being to yourself, you are practicing self-love. When you allow yourself to receive, you replenish yourself for better being and better giving.

Meaning comes from fulfillment, and fulfillment comes from following your own path, doing with your life what you really want to do and being who you are proud to be, rather than doing what you think you should do or being who you think you should be. Other people may need you, but *you* need you first. Maybe in your life, you take care of animals, or elders, or children, or people in need, or the planet. These are all beautiful, incredibly commendable works and we need people doing these things more than ever, but what if you gave yourself a little more time and care? This can create much more energy for you to give to your passions. Until you fulfill yourself, your actions toward others will deplete you rather than replenish you. You can get physically sick when you don't self-nurture. You could develop chronic pain, as I did, or get depressed, or crushed by panic attacks. Or the repercussions could be some form of burnout, when you can't even get basic things done or you don't feel any satisfaction or contentment in your life anymore.

A couple of years ago, I was working with one of my celebrity clients. She had just finished the first season of a new TV series, and everything was going great. The show was being nominated for awards, she was doing press interviews everywhere, and anyone looking at her from the outside would think her life was perfect. When it came time for her to fly back out to start filming the second season, leaving her husband, child, and household behind, she texted me because she didn't feel right. She was suddenly getting an outbreak of acne and she felt overwhelmed, anxious, angry, and torn between her work and her family life. The project she loved had lost all its joy and she said she felt that her stress level was a nine out of ten.

I talked with her for a while, and it was obvious that she was exhausted and suffering from burnout. She hadn't given herself any time to rest, recover, and receive while she was home. She kept on effort-ing when she had intended to relax. The first thing I had her do was to make a list of everything she had to do: Who required her time? When would she be on set? And what time slots did she have when there were no actual immediate demands on her? During these times, we scheduled in purposeful *not-doing* and rest. Just knowing she would have these pockets of not-doing helped her feel calmer and better about doing. Her days felt less overwhelming because she could now see that it would not be all work all the time. She could do what she needed to do, but also rejuvenate herself with periods of not-doing.

Sometimes the break you need is from people. It might be a demanding friend or your whole family. One of my friends feels a lot of obligation toward her family and she has had to make three divisions: her alone, her family as a separate entity apart from her, and the family as one unit of which she was an integrated part, with all the obligations and energy that involved. She recognized she had been spending all her time focusing on being an inextricable part of the family unit, without making time for herself as an individual, or allowing time for her family members to exist as individuals with their own relationships that don't involve her. She had to extricate herself just enough to regain her sense of her own identity.

Pay attention when your body goes on alert, gets exhausted, or loses joy. That is your intuition calling out to you to take care of yourself. Give yourself space to receive love so you can fill yourself up.

There is a time and a place to push and challenge yourself. Sometimes burning bright means living with an inner fire to experience what's possible for you, to push through the murkiness and the stagnation and the parts that don't want to bloom yet. But you also need to give yourself space for the growth, to explore and find your truth. There's no hurry. You don't have a deadline. This is life and it's messy and it's beautiful. You are living with a purpose right now, even if you don't know it yet. Rushing it and feeling anxious or having pain is not necessary in order to open up and receive all your life is waiting to offer you on this journey.

I was reading my horoscope the other day, and something it said rang true to me. It said that nature doesn't apologize for its seasons, for its dormant times and its burgeoning times. It doesn't apologize for its long cold nights or its radiant blooming days. It exists in its own time, regenerating in cycles. It does what it needs to do in its own natural cycles. And so can you. Give yourself what you need to regenerate and follow your own seasons.

THE DISCOMFORT OF JOY

A strange thing can happen when your life gets easier and feels better and you begin to have periods of joy and happiness. You may feel strangely uncomfortable in this new space. Why oh why, my love, would you feel bad about feeling good? I actually see this happen a lot. When you are used to living in a state of constant resistance, letting go can feel too easy, and then you start waiting for the other shoe to drop or for the rug to get pulled out from under you. You may not trust the good feeling, or you may just feel an underlying nervousness or even fear about a condition that feels so new to you.

Rather than just being present to receive and enjoy those moments of feeling good, people often try to find something bad, or even to sabotage their own happiness by dredging up an old imprint or negative thinking. Just as it takes practice to move through difficult feelings without efforting, it also takes some practice to move through good feelings without efforting, and with faith and trust in the rightness of your joy when you are blessed with it.

I've experienced this myself. I've had moments when things were shifting in positive ways, and at first I would think, "Wow, my life is so awesome!" But, soon after, my fear and my imprints would rise up and I'd think, "Kelsey, shouldn't you be doing something more? You're probably doing something wrong. You're going to mess this up if you make a mistake. You're going to lose all the good things if you don't try harder to hold on!" Then my mind would begin to manufacture drama. I might think, "Now that my career is going so well, I'm not being a good wife because I'm too busy," or "Now that I have this new opportunity, I'm afraid I might not be good enough to pull it off," or "My students or clients will probably be disappointed in me and my work," or "Now that everything's good, I'd better not let anything else change. I need to control this good luck!"

I make up all these stories to distract myself from how uncomfortable it can be to just sit in the moment and receive the beauty, peace, and joy of my life. The state of change brought up all my old imprints—obsession with productivity, fear of imperfection, guilt for not giving all of myself to others, or the belief that I'll never be enough. Your imprints and your fear will often jump in to remind you to be careful, to protect yourself, and to stay the same, even if "the same" is painful. But your fear is an adviser, not your director.

If your life is going great, you might think, "I really should be more stressed out right now—what am I not seeing?" or you may feel guilty that you aren't doing what you were doing before (like staying in a bad relationship or an unfulfilling job), even though it wasn't what you wanted to be doing. People can feel guilty about being happy or feeling free or having power when others aren't happy or don't feel free or don't have power. But these are imprints, too. You always have a choice. You don't have to run those old programs or feel guilty about aligning with your purpose and experiencing joy.

Sometimes this process can happen in disguise. For example, sometimes people in Los Angeles who do yoga, massage, meditation, and other spiritual practices can become obsessive about doing these things with extreme effort. They are using these restorative and healing practices in a way that is counterproductive to the very purpose of the practices. I see the same thing happening to people who are high achievers or who seem to have enormous amounts of public success. I've worked with many of them, and while some have grounding practices that do keep them in balance, many of them struggle with their obsession to control all aspects of their lives. This leaves them feeling anxiety, physical pain, insomnia, burnout, mental fatigue, addiction, and more. In both of these examples, people think they are evolving because of their success or their spiritual practices, but they've just dressed those same old imprints in a fancier costume.

Sometimes the only way to get out of this cycle is to just stop being so productive. Stop doing and stop trying so hard, and see how that feels. Never forget that you are a human being, not a human doing. Whenever you feel consumed with doing, remember that is not your true function. Check in with what your being needs in the moments when you're preoccupied with doing. How do you feel when you don't have any agenda and you don't have any to-do list? Do you feel uncomfortable without chaos, pain, lists, or obstacles? Sit with that feeling. Dig into it. Why do you think you feel so uncomfortable with ease? Give yourself time and space to feel the discomfort so you can bring awareness to any old imprints that are still active. If you feel discomfort, try not to lapse back into your hustle-and-grind mode. Stay with the rest, digest, and repair mode. Engage your parasympathetic nervous system and focus on finding gratitude for this moment of peace in your life. Ask yourself why you are fighting something you want.

When things are rough and there is chaos, pain, fear, obstacles, or overwhelm, sit with that feeling. When things change, sit with that fear. When things are good, sit with that discomfort. Resistance is the impulse, but surrender is the remedy. Have faith in who you came here to be, do your best at being you, and let the rest go. When you let go of all the chaos, you will be able to see why you are here in this life. You'll be able to find your purpose and start doing what you are meant to do and being who you are meant to be. It might be much easier and much healthier for you than you ever imagined.

CHECK-IN TIME:

Let's take a moment so that you can pause and check in with yourself. Take some deep breaths and focus inward. How are you feeling? Don't judge, just notice.

EXCAVATING
PURE JOY

CHAPTER FOUR

The Burning Bright Triad of Wholeness

Your mind is an entire world, your heart is an entire cosmos, and your soul is an entire universe.

—MATSHONA DHLIWAYO, ZIMBABWEAN PHILOSOPHER AND AUTHOR

W HEN YOUR BODY, mind, and spirit are aligned and synchronized, there will be so much joy available to you. In the next few chapters of the book, we're going to focus on how you can bring awareness and openness to your body, mind, and spirit, one by one. Body, mind, and spirit each exist on their own, but each is also connected to the others. These forces are one within you, and when they are in balance, you will be in balance.

When you begin to heal one part of the triad of wholeness, you may find that the other parts align. Alternatively, you may need to work on more than one part to feel balanced. A friend of mine who is a chiropractor tells me that she initially approached her work with her focus purely on the physical body, but she has come to see that her patients are more than their physical bodies—she can adjust them over and over again, but if they never address their emotions, they never get better. The pain her patients experienced wasn't so much neuromuscular as it was somatic-visceral, emotional pain manifested as physical pain. When she started talking to her patients about the stress aspect of healing, she started to get much better results. It changed her entire practice. In the same way, therapists who focus on mental health often find that their patients do better if they also begin taking better care of their physical bodies.

You can accelerate your healing by engaging all these parts of you. Body, mind, and spirit each reverberate with their own subtleties and sub-meanings, and every practice and philosophy I have ever studied—yoga, meditation, Reiki, emotional freedom technique (EFT, aka tapping), chakras—all involve balancing each of these elements.

Body, mind, and spirit are linked to certain basic aspects of life (these identifiers are based on my personal experiences with myself, my clients, and my students over the years):

- **BODY** encompasses your physical composition and structure, health, survival, basic needs, security, money, foundation, safety, work, and physical practices—like exercise, yoga, and food—plus physical contact with others, as well as your home and work environments and groundedness on the actual physical earth.

- **MIND** includes thoughts, feelings, emotions, issues like anxiety and depression, fear and grief, as well as skills like creativity and intellect. It also governs dreams, planning, analyzing, understanding, mindfulness, conversation with others, practices like EFT and meditation, and the mental connection to one's life purpose.

- **SPIRIT** includes nature, God, intuition, energy flow, relationships, love of self and love of others, problems like loneliness and isolation, connection to something higher than the individual, connection to the energy in other people and the community, spiritual practices like prayer, and healing energy work like Reiki.

Each aspect of this triad can be your focus for healing, depending on where you feel you need to start. If you focus on your body, you will gain health. If you focus on your mind, you will connect to your feeling of purpose. If you focus on your spirit, you will open to receiving support and love as part of relationships, trusting life, and building your community. Each one of these will nurture the others. You cannot be well in one without the others. These three basic human needs—health, purpose, and community, as they exist in your body, mind, and spirit—connect us all.

At a fundamental level as human beings, in order to feel a sense of belonging, love, capability, support, fulfillment, and peace, you need to:

1. **KNOW YOU CAN HEAL.** *Even if you have a chronic disease or some major health problem, working with body awareness and acceptance can help you to better understand the disease in your body so you can move into a state of acceptance, harmony, and love on your journey, no matter where you are. That is its own kind of medicine, to examine what you came here to learn and to give yourself permission to love yourself and your body the whole way through. I know from personal pain and experience that this may feel challenging, and I want you to know right now that every single part of you is worthy of healing. You are far more powerful as a healer of your own body than you think.*

2. **KNOW YOUR SENSE OF PURPOSE.** *Knowing that you came here for a reason and that every day has a purpose will help you to feel and understand why you are here. Working with your own*

thoughts and expressing your feelings more openly, even if just to yourself, can help you to define that purpose. It's okay if you don't know what your purpose is at this moment in life; that doesn't mean you don't have one. The more you keep showing up for yourself, and the more you continue to become aware of your thoughts and whether or not they are serving you, the more you will come into alignment with your purpose. Your purpose is innate and part of you. You will discover and connect to it more and more as you grow and open to your life's possibilities. Just continue to be open to all parts of yourself, in order to give your life a clearer sense of direction and meaning.

3. **KNOW YOU HAVE SUPPORT.** *Your spirit is connected by energy to the energies of others, as well as to a universal loving energy that brings us all together in the most sacred of unions. Understanding that you are and always have been connected to other people and to something higher will help you to feel more trust, faith, surrender, and sacred vulnerability in your life. It's essential to know that you are supported and worthy of that support. No matter how much you feel supported or not supported in this moment, others are seeking love and connection with you. The more you free yourself to receive that love and support, and the more you give your love and support to others, the more it will keep showing up in your life.*

Every person at any moment may have imbalances in all these areas, but most of us tend to have a primary problem in one of them. When you identify yours, you'll know where to start your work. As you begin to balance the area where you feel the most imbalanced, know that the other areas will begin to shift as well.

BODY: RESTORING HEALTH

Your physical body is your substance, and dis-ease at this level affects your physical health. This was my area of primary imbalance or, at least, it was the most obvious and unbearable imbalance in my own perception. Some signs that your primary imbalance may be in your body include:

- Chronic physical pain of any kind.

- Worrying you won't have enough energy to do or show up for your life.

- Lower back pain or pelvic pain, specifically near your root chakra (page 213).

- Any disease diagnosis.

- A lack of fitness—if exercising or moving vigorously through your life is difficult or seems impossible to you.

- Rapid weight gain or loss, and/or an inability to lose or gain weight, when this would be beneficial for your health.

- Eating disorders.

- A lack of passion, creativity, or sexual desire.

- Sleep and fatigue issues, either having trouble getting or staying asleep, or feeling tired during the day, even when you did get enough sleep.

- Clumsiness, dizziness, balance problems, or other feelings of not knowing where your body is in space.

- Allergies to elements of your environment, like pollen, dust, animals, or food.

- A feeling of a loss of connection with the natural world.

- A feeling of not being safe or secure.

- Hypochondria, now often called "somatic symptom disorder," or the feeling that something is always physically wrong with you, even if you aren't sure what it is.

- A fear that you won't be able to meet your basic physical needs, or a fear that you will lack sufficient resources (including money).

- A feeling that you aren't aware of your own body and its needs, or that you mostly exist in your mind or in your external activities. You may feel unsure of what to eat, how to move, and how to heal and nourish your body.

If this sounds like the area you feel you need to work on most, look to chapter 5, where you can dig deeper into this aspect of yourself and find practices that help to heal, balance, and restore your physical health. Then go to chapter 8, to find some body-focused rituals. The techniques you will learn will help you get back inside your body, release old physical imprints, and ground you in the present moment. Find that sense of rootedness, so you can reclaim safety and security in your body, even if it's not functioning as you wish it would.

~~~~

MIND: FINDING PURPOSE

The mental body is the realm of your thoughts. It contains all the things you think about, how you reason, how you process your feelings, how you take in information. You work out your purpose and your place on this planet with your mind. Your mind makes plans, visualizes your dreams, analyzes situations, and helps you figure out solutions to problems. Your mind is like the paper you write on to work through your thoughts. For many people, especially those who feel alienated from their physical bodies, the mind can become too dominant, but for others, the physical body dominates and the mind loses energy, clarity, and stimulation.

The mind is often subject to obsessive-compulsive behavior, fear, and control of any kind. Your imprints influence your thoughts, and your thoughts control your behaviors. Many of my students get stuck in mind loops, where they can't seem to escape the mental noise. Some experience mental imbalances in their physical bodies because chakras (page 213) are blocked. Signs that your mental state is out of balance might include:

- Anxiety, panic, nervousness.

- Feelings of chronic stress, never being able to relax.

- Feelings of burnout—inability to do simple daily life tasks, wishing you never had to work again or that you could run away from your life.

- Feelings of inadequacy, thinking you are not good enough or that you are "fooling everybody" into thinking you are competent.

- Low self-esteem, lack of confidence.

- Avoiding social activities because you don't feel like socializing.

- Excessive worry, obsessive negative thoughts.

- Chronic headaches, especially around your temples.

- Chronic digestive issues or "nervous stomach," primarily related to anxious feelings or self-confidence issues, especially around the solar plexus chakra (page 213).

- Chronic sore throat, around the throat chakra (page 213), especially if it coincides with problems verbally expressing yourself.

- Feelings of anger and irritation that seem out of proportion with the situation.

- Depression, sadness, feeling down, loss of joy in activities you used to find pleasurable.

- Trouble concentrating, brain fog, confusion.

- Mood swings.

- Insomnia from overthinking.

- Compulsive behavior—you can't control your eating, your spending, or what you say to other people.

- Feeling lost, directionless, not having a clear sense of what your purpose is.

- Substance abuse, addiction, or other self-harming behaviors.

If this sounds like the area where you feel most out of balance, you can go into more depth with your mind and find many practices, and exercises, that restore and harmonize the mind in chapter 6. In chapter 9, find rituals specifically for the mind. Working with your mind when you've got a lot of noise in there is about quieting and softening the noise, releasing stress and control, and bringing awareness to imprints. Meditation and emotional freedom technique (EFT, also sometimes called tapping) practices are some of the best mind-healers that exist because they help with awareness and release.

SPIRIT: CONNECTING WITH YOURSELF, OTHERS, AND A HIGHER POWER

The spiritual body is the seat of your soul. It is the part of you that connects with yourself, with other beings, with the unseen, with nature, and with something greater than yourself. Your spiritual body channels the energy that binds us all together at a spiritual level. For some people, this is the least familiar part of the body-mind-spirit triad, but getting to know this part of yourself better is a mystical and magical experience.

To bring this part of yourself into a state of flow and harmony with your physical body and your mind is to tune in to that energy or essence inside of you. This is the channel for intuiting and understanding things that aren't logical, but that you have a knowingness about. Spirit is where surrender happens, where trust in something bigger and greater for your life comes into play, and it is the mode through which you can let go and not need to *know* and *do* all the time. If you are losing energy in this part of yourself, some of the signs include:

- Feelings of personal isolation and loneliness.

- Feelings of denseness, blockage, stagnation.

- A disturbing sense that all things are separate and we are all alone in the universe.

- A deep longing for belonging and community.

- A loss of religious faith or spiritual beliefs you once had and feel a lack of now.

- Chronic headaches, especially centered in your forehead, near the third-eye chakra, or at the top of your head, around your crown chakra (page 213).

- Chest pain around your heart chakra (page 213).

- Feelings of selfishness, specifically not caring about anyone else but yourself.

- Not dealing with or not letting go of the pain from the loss of a loved one or the end of a relationship.

- Materialism, obsession with always wanting more things.

- Social media addiction.

- Not feeling that you know who you are, identity crisis.

- Feeling as if nobody really cares about you or loves you.

- Feeling that life has no meaning.

- A sense of doom or fear that you can't pin down.

- An overwhelming fear of death.

- A lack of compassion for other human beings, animals, the earth, or our world community.

- A lack of desire to share yourself and your gifts and your love with the world. This can manifest as not feeling the desire or not feeling the ability to be part of the world and its beauty.

To nourish your spiritual side, open up to allow energy to move and flow through your body and mind, as well as in and out of you from beyond the physical limits of your body. Feeling and receiving this expansive life-force energy is the way to access your ability to connect to a deeper part of your soul. The more you work with this vibration, the better you will be able to feel the energy of other people, animals, even inanimate objects (especially in nature, like rocks, trees, and water). This invisible energy is what knits all three of your parts together: body to mind to spirit, unified into *you*. In chapter 7, you'll learn more about spirit and how you can access and strengthen yours, as well as guidance for reconnecting with others and regaining a sense of community and a spiritual practice. You'll also find do-it-yourself energy techniques, including Reiki, of course, but also some others. In chapter 10, you'll find some rituals designed for spiritual nourishment.

HOW TO USE THE REST OF THIS BOOK

The next three chapters in this book contain a lot of information about the body, mind, and spirit in general, which you can use to find your own disharmonies so you can clear, heal, and begin to excavate the pure joy you came here to live and receive. Even if you have a primary dysfunction in one part, I hope you will read all the chapters because you may discover other ways you can grow and begin to allow for joy you may have never known was available to you.

As you read the rest of this book, also know that not all the information will resonate with you, and not every practice will be right for you, so take the ones that you feel a sense of connection with, and start there. This book contains its own vibration of healing for you, and its own magic intended to support you. There is distance Reiki (Reiki sent across space and/or time) infused into this book just for you, and it is meant to have its own wisdom to support and guide you, so you can communicate with it. As you come back to this book over the course of weeks, months, or even years, you may find that other practices you weren't interested in before suddenly jump out at you when you are ready for them. That is just as it is intended to be.

After you've made your way through this book, you may find that you can just open it to a random page and find something you were meant to receive for that specific day. I also want you to feel the freedom to play around in this book by skipping from place to place, subject to subject, practice to practice, if you have that impulse. You don't need to do it all in order. You don't have to be rigid and structured, unless that is your way and it feels right for you right now. Trust that this book will manifest in your life and co-create with you in whatever way best serves you on that day and in that moment.

This is the time to recommit to a level of self-love and curiosity that will keep you involved in this work. This is the time for you to start exercising your intuitive powers and listening to your own body, mind, and spirit, to discover what it is you need to find your own sense of wholeness. Please, my dear, love yourself enough that you are ready and willing to take responsibility for the one divine, amazing, magical life you have been gifted. This is the time to remember you have an incredible, sacred inner knowing, and you are able to heal from within. You are your greatest teacher. You have access to all you need to burn bright. Have faith that you can!

And always remember that your goal is not to be perfect. We are all imperfect. The goal is to allow yourself your imperfections while also allowing your wholeness to come into its most full manifestation, with body, mind, and spirit in harmony, bound by the flow, movement, and grace of divine energy through every aspect of yourself and your life. Even on a day when you feel filled with physical pain, or grief, or loss, or anger, or anxiety, or any other negative feeling, remember to breathe through it and know that you don't need to change it. Feel it and it will pass. To move beyond it, let go of your efforts to control that pain or strong feeling or reality check. It might feel unbearable for a moment, but bearing the unbearable is as much a part of life as celebrating the most joyful moments. Sometimes the greatest pain is exactly what brings about the greatest gifts.

Finally, as you navigate through these chapters, moving inward and working with your energy, remember that, within you, there is nothing to fix. There is nothing to change. All the work in this book is in the service of being present with yourself in each moment and from that place, listening and hearing where you are and what is happening inside you and what you need next. Choose to feel. Choose to live. These practices are not meant to be curative, but rather to serve your highest good, bringing you into awareness of your own human experience, your natural rhythms, your needs, desires, and feelings. Lean into your truth and love on it so you can become one with it.

One of the things I say in my workshops is, "If there was anything we weren't meant to feel, it wouldn't exist." That means all your grief, pain, sadness, burnout, vulnerability, fear, aloneness, and worry are just as valid and important to experience as your joy, excitement, love, vibrancy, connection, passion, support, and sense of community. It's all part of the beauty of being human, and jumping right into all that mess means jumping into your own unlimited potential to shine.

CHAPTER FIVE

The Burning Bright Body

Every realm of nature is marvelous.
—ARISTOTLE, ANCIENT GREEK PHILOSOPHER

YOUR BODY IS your rock. You rely on it to get you through this life. This is the first part of the triad of wholeness—body harmony is a foundation on which you can build mental and spiritual harmony, vitality, and fullness. If health is your challenge, this is the place for you to start. For others, it may be more useful to start with mind before body or spirit, or to start with spirit to connect to body and mind. But I want to start with the body because when you hurt physically or do not have physical health, it's hard to feel or find anything else. You might be able to push through for a while, but at some point—like that morning I woke up and couldn't move my neck—it's going to stop you.

Whether you have a diagnosis or you just don't feel as vital, strong, or healthy as you could, there are profound practices that can restore balance and harmony to the rock that is your body. The earth is its own kind of body and it is the foundation under our feet. It also has medicine for the body. Being out in nature helps the body to feel more grounded, and the earth provides us with real whole food, oxygen from trees, plant medicine, sunshine, healing water, soil, and rock to help ground us, including crystals to direct and focus energy. This chapter is about tuning in to your physical body to find the healing connection between your body and the earth for physical wholeness, and to plug the body back in to the triad of wholeness so it harmonizes and connects with the mind and the spirit.

~~~~

YOUR HEALTH STATE

As a society, we need healing. People are experiencing chronic disease at rates beyond anything we have ever seen in the history of the world. According to the CDC,[1] 6 out of 10 adults in the United States currently have a chronic disease, and 4 out of 10 have two or more chronic diseases. Autoimmune diseases, chronic fatigue syndrome, thyroid disease (like Hashimoto's), diabetes, high blood pressure, high cholesterol, heart disease, cancer, lung disease, kidney disease, stroke . . . 1 in 3 Americans has prediabetes, people are having heart attacks and strokes at much younger ages (often in their thirties and forties), 50 million Americans have an autoimmune disease,[2] obesity is at an all-time high at 39.8 percent of US adults, and almost 75 percent of US adults are overweight. Only 1 in 10 adults eats the number of fruit and vegetable servings recommended by the government's dietary guidelines[3] (which are most likely not nearly enough).

Autoimmune diseases, like Hashimoto's in particular, seem to be plaguing my students and clients. From an energetic perspective, I see these physical health problems as consequences of burnout. When you are overwhelmed, anxious, and not living your joy, and when you are stressed all the time, your body can begin to break down and your immune system suffers. Chronic diseases may be the end result. But you are not a public health statistic and only you can know if your health needs more of your attention. Take some time to tune in to your body and its messages. What do you feel is right for you right now? Engage your intuition. Maybe you feel drawn to trying a yoga class, or acupuncture, or you would really love a massage. Maybe you are curious about Reiki, or you just want to do something simple, like cook healthy food at home more often, or just drink a full glass of water with lemon first thing every morning, or sit quietly for five minutes in the evening before you go to sleep, to settle your mind. Maybe you feel drawn to walking for ten minutes a few times a week, but that's all you can handle right now.

Everything you do for your body will cause a shift. Even if you just visualize how you will look and feel when your body is healthy and you feel in harmony with the world around you, seeing it leads you toward being it. All the tiny changes you make for yourself and your health can turn into life-changing transformations.

Open your consciousness with intention for healing, and shifts and opportunities will come to you. Look for universal signs throughout your day and week that you are on the right track. If you're working on your health, you might see a poster announcing that the farmers' market starts this weekend, or that there will be a free community yoga class in the park, or that a local meditation center is having evening meditation sessions. You might be driving down a street you haven't been on before and notice a new park or a trailhead calling to you, or get a sudden urge to go to the beach and put your feet in the sand. Honor those signs and impulses you feel within yourself. Maybe someone tells you about how they have started riding their bike instead of driving to work and you can see yourself doing that. Maybe you pass by a fresh fruit stand you've never noticed before on the way home from work, or someone gives you the name of a great functional medicine doctor, or you find out that a local hiking group explores the natural areas outside your city every Saturday. These aren't coincidences. They are beacons. The direction is out there. When you start looking, you will start seeing. And one of the most important things to see is how you are showing up to take care of your body, which is your temple.

PHYSICAL INTUITION

Many of the sections in this chapter are about using your intuition to determine how to take care of your own health in ways that can guide you toward the right foods, movements, and practices. Physical intuition can also guide you toward what to put in your interior space and also what to do and feel when you are outside in nature.

Overall, physical intuition is a type of intuition you can refine and practice using, so you can get better and better at it. You can integrate this practice into your morning routine, or tune in to yourself anytime you start to feel the tension of stress rising in your chest by checking in with yourself throughout the day and asking yourself what your physical body needs.

When you take responsibility for what is happening inside your physical body and honor it no matter where you are or what you are doing, you will bring your physical body back into harmony with the rest of your wholeness. Whether you are at home alone, feeling stressed at work, or waiting to see a doctor, give yourself permission to listen within, then speak your truth to yourself and to those who care for you, so you can get what you need for the rock that is your body.

WHEN WAS YOUR LAST CHECKUP?

One way to bring awareness to your body and its health state is to see a doctor for a physical and get basic tests run, like a blood panel, cholesterol, blood pressure, blood sugar, thyroid function, or whatever else your doctor recommends for you. If everything is normal, that's great—now you have a baseline and you can watch for trends at every yearly physical. If something is out of normal range, now you know and you can do something about it.

The sooner you address any health issues, the easier it will be to bring them back into balance. Even though it is my experience that imprints can contribute to health issues, it is always a good idea to get the medical perspective—it can be life-saving! For a long time, I would let the doctors just take my blood and then I would get a voice mail, saying everything looked good. I never asked questions and I never asked to see my numbers or results. I just took their word for it that I was okay. Then I found out what happened to my friend Mina. Mina thought she was healthy, but she had just turned fifty and her younger sister had already had a heart attack at age forty-five. Mina was healthy and fit, but she thought, Hey, why not know more? She asked her doctor for some additional tests, including a cardiac test for inflammation. When her results came back, she found out that her inflammation was so high that she was in the high-risk category for a heart attack!

Mina wasn't overweight, she exercised, and she ate well, or so she thought, but she had a high-stress job and she had a lot of anxiety. Her cholesterol and blood pressure were normal, but her doctor said she had to switch to an anti-inflammatory diet and start practicing stress management immediately. If she hadn't thought about her risk factors and asked for additional tests, she never would have found out. She began meditating regularly, delegated some of her job responsibilities to others, shifted to a more plant-based diet, and started exercising less intensely. Her inflammation is now almost back to normal, but that never would have happened if she hadn't paid attention and asked questions. If you aren't getting the kind of response from your doctor that you want, you might look into a functional medicine doctor. They are typically much more willing to do more extensive labwork to give you an even more detailed idea of where you are health-wise. Whether or not you feel you have an intuitive connection to your body and its state of health, getting your bloodwork done is a great place to start to see your numbers and make necessary changes to your lifestyle.

So get outside. Plant your feet on the ground. Touch the trees, plants, and flowers. Breathe the air. Feel the sun, wind, rain. Find the energy and power in earth, water, fire, and air. Eat real whole food that the earth provides. Participate in the natural world in whatever way you can. Honor your body. Protect your health. Move. Breathe. Sleep. And live. Taken as a whole, the body and the earth are physical manifestations of energy, incarnated in this present moment. Finding the union within your own body, so that you feel grounded, strong, brave, and clear, will help you to understand and feel the energy that connects your physical body to this magnificent rock that holds and supports us as it spins us around the sun. This is how to discover the ultimate harmony of the visceral, tangible, beautiful level of physical existence.

~~~~

PHYSICAL CHECK-IN

Do this exercise whenever you feel you need to get a read on how your physical body is doing and what it might need, especially if you feel you need something, but you aren't sure what it is.

Find a comfortable position, either sitting or lying down. Every part of your body should feel supported. Be quiet and breathe naturally for a minute or so, until you begin to feel a sense of inner calm. When you feel ready, ask yourself: "Is there anything I need to do for myself right now?"

Don't jump to a response or think about what you should do or have to do. This is not about obligation or guilt. Instead, just listen for a response from deep within your physical body. It might take a few minutes. Be patient. Just wait, breathe, and listen.

Eventually, you might begin to get a visual image, or hear a voice, or just have a feeling. It might be telling you that you need to get up and take a ten-minute walk outside, or play some soft music and just close your eyes and listen for ten minutes. If you are at work, maybe you need to get up and do a lap around the building or climb up and down a flight of stairs before you go back to your desk, or step outside for a few deep breaths of fresh air and some sunshine on your skin. Maybe you really need to eat something. Maybe you need to do a few gentle yoga poses, or splash cold water on your face.

Be open to whatever messages come through. The better you get at listening, the better you will get at hearing. What you need can change from moment to moment, so don't try to predict it. Just rely on your body wisdom to tell you. Are you hungry? Tired? Restless? Do you hurt? Do you feel joyful? Honor that.

When you feel that you have an answer, sit with the answer for a few minutes, then slowly open your eyes. If you can, respond to your body's call right away. If you can't, make a plan for when you can do what you feel you need to do for yourself as soon as possible.

<hr />

INTUITIVE OR MINDFUL EATING

There are a million ways to eat, and a thousand ways to eat a healthy diet, but the one I like the most is intuitive eating. To me, this is the most natural way to commune with food because you use your intuition to ask your body what it needs and you listen well enough that you hear the answers that come from deep within, rather than from the external cues that convince so many people to eat what isn't good for them, or to eat too much or too often. You don't need a diet plan and you don't need to count anything as long as you focus on mostly whole foods from the earth, and you listen to your own intuition about what to eat and how much and when. Your own body knows better about what it needs than any advertisement or best-selling book or diet doctor or social media post or friend who thinks they know what everyone should be eating.

For people who are used to dieting or carefully tracking every calorie, carb, or fat gram, intuitive eating may feel scary. It is a leap of faith, for sure. At first you might not always be sure what is a craving and what is an intuition, but the more you work on fine-tuning your body awareness and the way you feel after following your intuition, the more you will understand the true nature of your body's messages about what you need. Some days you might feel as if all you want is fresh raw vegetables and juicy fruits. Other days you may feel a deep need for more protein or fat. Maybe you eat meat, but your body tells you that it's time to go vegetarian for a while, or maybe you are a vegetarian and your body tells you, every now and then, that it's time for a little bit of animal protein (either way, it's your body and your choice). If you have been diagnosed with a chronic condition such as an autoimmune disorder, following an anti-inflammatory diet can be life-changing. Part of intuitive eating is also giving your body what it needs to find balance and harmony. For you, this could look like increasing your intake of anti-inflammatory food, to help alleviate chronic stress in the body.

Your imprints can get in the way of intuitive eating, telling you things as simple as "You don't like broccoli" or as insidious as "You don't deserve dessert." But sometimes you might not be sure. The word *should* is usually a good clue, and here's why. There is a big difference between: "I *should* eat some vegetables" and "I feel like I *need* a big salad," or "I really *shouldn't* have any cake" and "I feel like a few bites of chocolate cake would *bring me joy* right now." Remember that fear and imprints tell you what you *should* and *shouldn't* do, but the body tells you what you need and deeply desire, not so you can hide or smother a bad feeling, but because it can help to balance and harmonize you.

Intuitive eating may not work for everyone, but some research reveals that eating based on external cues isn't helpful. One study showed that, in women, people who focused on label reading and nutrition facts were 17 percent more likely to binge eat.[4] Another study showed that college students who frequently weighed themselves and counted calories were more likely to have eating disorders than those who didn't do these things. The study concluded that promoting intuitive eating might improve college student health.[5] Another study that looked at the results of many different studies on mindful and intuitive eating determined that mindfulness is effective at addressing binge eating, emotional eating, and eating based on external cues, especially in people who were overweight, and that encouraging mindful eating might be helpful in general for weight management.[6]

Eating is a very common response to anxiety, and disordered eating, like binge eating, is often thought to be caused by anxiety.[7] Like a drug, food can dull strong feelings and distract you. Mindfulness and focus on your own intuition can help you discern whether your perception of hunger has been sparked by anxiety, fear, unhappiness, procrastination, or any other distraction as opposed to genuine physical hunger. (Remember that you now know a lot more about why it's beneficial to feel your feelings.)

My very dear friend Susan grew up in a household where she felt she wasn't able to express herself or be heard by her family members. As with my family, Susan's family wasn't comfortable talking about emotions. Even when her sister had a near-suicide attempt in high school, nobody in the family wanted to talk about it, and after a few half-hearted therapy sessions, nobody mentioned it again. Susan knew this wasn't a healthy environment for her, so she went out of state for college as soon as she could.

Yet, the imprints lingered. As a child, sugary junk foods were often available and they were comforting. In her twenties, Susan struggled with bingeing on food and eating a lot of sugar because she thought it made her "happy," even though she was depriving her body of nutrient-rich food. When she was recently diagnosed with Hashimoto's disease (an autoimmune thyroid condition), Susan recognized that reaching for junk food and sugar in an effort to feel happy was a sort of attack on her own body, and that is just what an autoimmune disease does—your immune system attacks your own body. Even though Susan eats pretty well now, she still struggles with indulgences for emotional comfort. I talked about this with her and she realized that she wasn't listening to the voice of her higher self when making food choices. Now she has committed to looking at food as something to heal her, rather than to fill an emotional void, and as triggers come up, she sees them as learning opportunities, rather than excuses to indulge.

Sugar is a trigger for many people because it makes life feel "sweeter," emotionally, even though, of course, it doesn't solve anything. My mom had crazy sugar addictions—whenever our family went out to dinner, she would ask for the dessert menu before we even got the dinner menu and then the first thing she would ask the waiter was "What's the best dessert you have?" I was always so embarrassed as a kid, and even as an adult. Looking back, I suspect that she wasn't really hungry for dessert. Maybe she was filling a void inside herself with something sweet, so she could feel good for a little while. Maybe she didn't even realize that's what she was doing.

If you ever read diet books, you've probably heard the old quote by Hippocrates, the father of modern medicine: "Let food be thy medicine and medicine be thy food." This is how I try to think of food. Will this thing I want to eat be healing for my body? Food is not an antidepressive or an anti-anxiety medicine. When you use it to make you happy, it is a temporary fix, a bandage over a bad feeling. If you eat to bury your strong feelings, you are just covering them up, not curing them.

Over the many years I've been working with clients, I see over and over again how people eat when they are truly happy and fulfilled as opposed to how they eat when they are depressed, burned out, insecure, overwhelmed, guilt-ridden, sad, lonely, anxious, or unfulfilled. All these feelings can impact your ability to eat intuitively because these feelings may be louder than your intuition. It's essential to feel the feelings and to get through them, but notice if they are triggering you to care for yourself with nourishing food, or to hurt yourself physically with empty or excessive food. When you are going through a difficult time in your life, it is even more important to nourish yourself and give your body the love and support it needs to love and support you.

Look at the overall level of joy and happiness in your life now and in the past, and see if that coincides with how you choose or have chosen to eat. When you can't hear your intuition and you feel the compulsion to drown out your feelings with sugar or alcohol or potato chips, that is your cue to go in exactly the opposite direction. Intuitive eating is a very beautiful and simple practice, but it can also be difficult if you've been separated from your joy and alienated from yourself for a while.

✦ PLANNING FOR ✦ THE TOUGH TIMES

When you're going through hard times, it's helpful to follow a more regimented eating plan—a "When I can't hear my intuition, I will choose to eat XYZ" kind of plan—that you create ahead of time. Use it in those periods when you know you need nutrition but might not always be in the right frame of mind to make good decisions about what to eat. For you, that might mean whole foods only, or that you will not eat sugary or fried food, or that you will take a break from alcohol. Whatever you know your weak spot is, balancing it can be your contingency plan, until you can hear your inner voice again. All the while, though, keep checking in with yourself and listening. Your intuition is *always* there, and the human body has the ability to heal itself, but there are times when each of us needs a support system to give us the strength to follow our intuition. Other supports you could use in difficult times might include a therapist, a nutritionist, a dietitian, or a support group.

Another very simple tool you can use as you navigate intuitive eating is the pause. This means pausing before you go into that moment of bingeing. This also works for any kind of compulsive behavior you might struggle with, like shopping or drinking alcohol. Just take a moment before you do that thing you find it hard *not* to do, and ask yourself: Is this thing I'm about to do filling some emptiness in me? What really goes in that space? Truthfully, when you feel happy, content, and satisfied, you usually don't feel the need to take in more. If you can figure out something that would be more fulfilling than the cookie or the glass of wine or the shoes, see if you can make a shift and try that thing, like writing in your journal or taking a walk or doing a few yoga poses or meeting your friend to talk something out. Even if you do go on to eat or buy or do the thing, at least you will do so mindfully, having asked yourself the questions.

When you are in a place where you feel stronger and more joyful, and your intuition seems to be back online, you can go back to your intuitive eating practice. Whether you are trying to lose or gain weight right now or you just want to feel healthy, intuitive eating might be exactly what can help you get back in touch with your body. Here is an exercise to practice intuitive eating.

INTUITIVE EATING EXERCISE

I'm someone who loves to eat. I will regularly have a pizza with my kids or a dinner out with friends with wine and dessert, but I also know when my body is craving clean, natural food or I need a break from overindulging. Sometimes I can tell I just need to keep things simpler. I've learned to do this through intuitive eating. Here's how you can try this natural way of tuning your relationship with food.

Every time you are ready to eat, sit quietly for a moment before eating even one bite. Remind yourself there is no rush. Close your eyes. Focus on your breath. Get to a calm space, then gently ask your body: *What is the best meal for my body right now?*

Wait for the answer. You might also ask: *Will this food nourish me right now?* Wait for the answer. Remind yourself that there is no rush. When you have an answer, open your eyes and, maintaining a feeling of inner peace and calm, prepare your meal.

If the answer is that you don't need food right now, ask your body: *What do I really need or want right now?* You may feel that your mind wants a distraction from something you've been procrastinating about or don't want to do, you're seeking some sort of reward, or you are trying to avoid facing or admitting to a feeling. Notice what it feels like beneath that false hunger. If you determine that the cause is something other than real hunger, stay in this place of focus and self-care. Let yourself take time to find an answer. Do you need to feel a feeling instead of pushing it down?

This is something to work on over time. It might feel difficult at first, but know that whenever you give in to the urge to eat when you aren't really hungry—but just don't want to feel your feelings—you will reinforce the message that food is an emotional crutch, rather than the beautiful, vibrant source of physical energy it really is. Instead of eating when you aren't hungry, turn to any of the practices in this or the next two chapters (or any of the rituals in part 3).

EXERCISE AND MOVEMENT

Bodies are built to move. A healthy body with good circulation, strong muscles, and limber joints gets and stays that way through movement. You might not need a lot of movement in your life. Or maybe you do. Maybe you thrive on super-intense movement or, maybe for you, intense exercise feels stressful and counterproductive. Natural body movement is meant to feel good and joyful, not obsessive, excessive, stress-inducing, burnout-promoting, or hyper-productive. People can get addicted to exercise and become chronic overexercisers, just as they can get addicted to food and become chronic overeaters. This is where your intuition comes into play again. When you get quiet and ask your body how it needs to move, it will tell you. Intuitive, mindful movement, according to what your body wants and needs, will help to defuse stress, rather than causing it or making it worse.

We know, based on many years of research studies, that regular exercise can reduce or even eliminate some of the physical changes that come with aging. And, it makes you feel better. I like to quote Elle Woods (played by Reese Witherspoon) in the movie *Legally Blonde*, who said that her fitness star client couldn't possibly be a murderer because "Exercise gives you endorphins and endorphins make you happy, and people who are happy just don't kill someone." Ha, I think that's true!

Only you can determine, through your own body communication, how much movement and what kind of movement are right for you at any given stage in your life. Remember that your imprints will tell you what you *should* do. If you think, "I really *should* go to the gym right now" or "I *should* get up off this couch and go for a walk," that is your fear, or your guilt, or your imprints talking. Messages that come genuinely from your body will sound more like this: "I feel like I need to get outside and take a walk right now with some healing fresh air" or "I feel like going to the gym in order to work out some of this stress energy" or "I'm exhausted, and I need to go take a nap or go to the spa for an afternoon to rest and allow myself to receive what I need." Your body will tell you what will help to bring it into balance and harmony without trying to force you to do something through guilt or anxiety. As you are deciding what you need, it may be helpful to know that there are three basic types of exercise:

1. *Cardiovascular exercise that gets your heart rate up.*

2. *Strength training that keeps muscles strong.*

3. *Stretching that keeps connective tissue and joints flexible.*

On any given day, you might do them all, or only one of them . . . or none of them. You can fulfill all three of these physical needs in endless ways—walking, running, dancing, cycling, weight lifting, yoga, Pilates. You can get all your movement through natural means, like walking, playing, hiking, going on bike rides with your family, playing recreational sports, or—my personal favorite—dancing for fun. Or you can be more structured and go to a gym, taking classes or using weight machines, if that's what brings your body joy. Some people love to exercise on a schedule, while other people don't like to plan. They move when they feel the urge to move.

To me, there is a difference between resting mindfully and lying on the couch and knowing full well that your imprints and fear are trying to keep you stuck there. Then there are times when you know you've drained everything you have to give and it's a much better idea for you to take a warm and healing bath, to read a book you love, and to get to sleep early.

Everyone is different, but if you are looking for a general guideline, the American Heart Association advises that most people get a total of 150 minutes of exercise a week. How you do that, though, is more flexible than we once thought. Recent research shows that it doesn't matter if you get it in fifteen 10-minute sessions or two 75-minute sessions each week, or in any other combination. You could do 30 minutes five days a week, or 50 minutes three days a week, or all 150 minutes in a single morning. (The 150 minutes is a minimum—you may want to do more, or even a bit less.)

A friend of mine is a district attorney and she came to me because she was feeling as if she really needed more exercise in her life.

Her husband is a lawyer, and they have two little boys. She spends her days taking bad guys off the streets and her Monday through Friday is pretty much booked from the moment she wakes up to the moment her head hits the pillow. But she wasn't feeling great. In the past, when she used to exercise more, she told me she felt a lot better in her body, and she wanted me to help her figure out how she could incorporate more movement into her life. But this was a real challenge—we were both having trouble figuring out how she could fit exercise in without having to get up at 3:30 every morning!

I'd always thought that daily, consistent exercise was the best way to make a difference in health, but I had just read this study that said working out for three or four hours on the weekend is just as good as working out every day. We figured out that she could work out for two hours on Saturdays, and for another hour or two on Sunday afternoon. That's all she needed to do for the week, and, because it was the weekend, she was often able to involve her family by choosing to do fun, active group activities with her husband and kids, like long bike rides or hikes. She and her husband also started doing a candlelight yoga class together as a date night on Friday evenings and went to dinner afterward. Problem solved.

Saving exercise for the weekends can really take the pressure off. If you constantly feel stressed and guilty because you haven't been using your gym membership or you can't even get outside for a daily walk, think about how you could move more with less pressure and without worrying that you have to do it every day. This flexibility helps to bypass the *should* so you can find joy in moving when you can.

Sometimes the healthiest practice is to go outside of a gym and into nature with all its healing and majesty. As Henry David Thoreau said: "There are moments when all anxiety and stated toil are becalmed in the infinite leisure and repose of nature."

A massage may seem like a luxury, but the benefits of massage and other forms of bodywork (like neuromuscular therapy, myofascial release, trigger point therapy, reflexology, and craniosacral therapy) have been well studied. Massage effectively reduces symptoms of anxiety, depression, and anger, and decreases heart rate and blood pressure. It's also great for relieving muscle strain and chronic pain, and inducing relaxation.[8] Because there are so many types of bodywork, you might need to experiment to find a style and a therapist you like, but once you do, the regular and consistent practice can be a supportive way to manage physical and mental health. If you do decide to try bodywork, however, don't forget the emotional part of your healing. Remember that the body supports the mind and the mind supports the body.

THE UNION OF YOGA

One of the most versatile and beneficial mind-body-spirit exercises you can do is yoga. Yoga may include cardiovascular exercise (as with vinyasa flow), strength training (lifting your own body weight), and, of course, stretching and flexibility training. It can also create space in the mind and feed your spirit, thanks to focused breathwork and body movement and still moments, especially during rest in savasana and through meditation.

To learn yoga and start practicing it regularly, you could take a yoga class, or do yoga at home out of a book or by following a video, or you could do intuitive yoga, once you know a few basics, by moving in whatever way you feel your body wants to move. Kate is one of my students who likes to incorporate intuitive yoga into her morning routine. She wakes up, meditates for five minutes, does some Reiki on herself, then lets that spiritual immersion guide her into some intuitive yoga on her yoga mat. She spends about forty-five minutes on this every morning and it puts her body and mind in a calm, centered place for the whole day.

Because yoga works with the flow in the body (just as acupuncture, Reiki, and other energy therapies do), it is one of the best ways to bring all the parts of the body into more unified wholeness, as *yoga* literally can be translated as "union." There are many styles of yoga, from easy and relaxing to challenging and vigorous. Almost all of us can find a style we like and enjoy, but as with any other movement, yoga should not be about dogmatic hyper-productivity. It shouldn't add more stress to your life. It should relieve stress and create a sense of unity between you and your body.

For you, that might mean an intensive daily practice because that makes you feel better and helps you manage the stress of your day. Or, you might do much better with some simple stretching and flowing movements because anything more intense makes you feel more stressed. It could be something just once or twice a week or a different type of practice each day. You have your own inner rhythm that relates to and interacts with the rhythms out there in the world. Honor your rhythm, and you will know exactly how to move. It might be yoga. It might not be yoga. What matters is that it's right for you, and feels good to your body.

Another powerful stress-relieving technique is the ancient practice of sound bathing. Sound bathing balances the nervous system and regulates the flow of energy within and through the body, and it can also be a powerful way to release emotions you haven't allowed yourself to feel. To try a sound bath, find a practitioner who can guide you. Experienced practitioners can actually switch you from a stress state (sympathetic nervous system) to a relax-and-repair state (parasympathetic nervous system) purely through the vibrations from sound.

Typically, in a session, you will lie down and the practitioner will play sounds on instruments, such as singing bowls, gongs, or bells, or play special music with certain vibrations and frequencies. You can feel the sounds actually reverberating and vibrating through your body. Afterward, you will likely feel calm, centered, and peaceful. Taking regular sound baths can be an effective way to keep your energy flowing and balanced.

NATURAL SLEEP HYGIENE

I used to have a lot of anxiety about sleep. I would worry about not getting enough, about not having gotten enough, and about what sleep deprivation might mean for my upcoming day. Would I have enough energy? Would I be exhausted and miserable that whole day? Was I going to get a headache because I didn't sleep? My worrying about it probably made my sleep deprivation feel worse than it would have felt if I hadn't anticipated so many problems from it. The stress of not sleeping and the stress of worrying about not sleeping would often make my neck hurt.

When your sleep patterns are off, that is a sign from your body that something needs attention. It could be the first sign you get that you are experiencing burnout, and getting good-quality sleep is an important way to support your body when you have burnout. One of the things that helped me to finally find peace surrounding sleep was to start intuiting and trusting my body's natural rhythms— sometimes I actually need less sleep, and sometimes I need more— and also to create a sleep ritual and practice it every night, whenever I could. At one point I received hypnosis for sleep because my anxiety had become overwhelming with upcoming travel to foreign countries where I would be leading workshops and teaching classes. We worked a lot on what was behind the energy of my fears about sleep, which was incredibly helpful. Also, because my husband snores, I didn't realize how much that was causing me to feel fearful right before falling asleep. I was waiting to see if his snores would wake me up. Through hypnosis and talking through some things directly with my husband, I was able to let go of the grip of this anxiety a bit, and not let it take over my mind and body.

When you do the same calming things every night, your body learns that those cues mean sleep is coming, so you begin to expect sleep and fall asleep more easily. You may have different things that work for you, but my sleep ritual includes turning off all TV and electronics one or two hours before going to bed. I make myself a cup of herbal tea and then I journal out all my thoughts from the day, so that when I go to bed, any lingering worries and concerns have been dumped out onto a piece of paper and I don't have to bring them to bed with me. Sometimes I read, but only things that make me feel peaceful, not excited or too intrigued to stop reading (like with a suspense novel). Last of all, I spend some time praying or meditating, then I lie down and Reiki myself.

Your routine might include a skin-care routine, or a gentle yoga routine, or laying out your clothes for the next day and packing your lunch. It doesn't have to be deep or spiritual. Anything that helps you to slow down the rhythm of your body works. Or, see page 249 for one of my favorite sleep rituals.

✦ CBD OIL FOR CALMING ✦

For some people, CBD oil, or cannabidiol oil, which is an oil de-rived from the cannabis or marijuana plant, can be therapeutic for calming and preparing for sleep. It has definitely helped me to relax. I take an organic, natural brand that doesn't con-tain THC (the psychoactive compound in marijuana that gets you "high"), and I take it in the late afternoon or early evening. It gently turns off my "doing" and turns on my rest-and-repair mode. (By the way, as of this writing, CBD without THC is cur-rently legal under federal law as long as it doesn't have any therapeutic claims on the label, although some state and city laws prohibit it.)[9] It's not for everyone, but for those who do use it, it can be very helpful.

EARTH AWAKENING

As public health is burning out, so is the health of our planet. The earth is our mirror and we can see our own health decline in the envi-ronmental crisis. The earth is a body that supports our physical bod-ies. To heal the earth is to heal ourselves, and to heal ourselves is to heal the earth. We are bound up with earth energy and the connec-tion goes both ways; humans have been connecting with earth energy for thousands of years. The earth has always had medicine for us, and we have the power within ourselves to give good medicine and energy back to the planet.

Developing earth awareness will help you to connect to the earth for healing. Think about your relationship to the planet. Do you notice the ground under your feet? Do you feel the air, the sun, the water, and the plants and trees in your immediate environment? Do you ever take time to get outside, taking a walk or a hike or just looking with attention at the natural world around you? It's easy to go through life distracted, only looking at computer, phone, and television screens, without really opening your eyes to your physical environment.

Every time you step outside and look around, try to notice the pockets of nature around you. If you can, smell the flowers and touch the plants you have around you during the day. Bring a new plant or fresh flowers inside your home. These parts of nature emit vibrations and they can connect to your natural rhythms to support you and your well-being. If you're outside, notice what plant life springs up through the cracks in the pavement, what trees shade your street, how the sun feels, whether the day is windy, cloudy, or clear. See if you can take a walk in a park, spend some time in a garden, or go on a hike. Research shows that looking at the color green can actually improve physical health, mental function, relationships, and the general feeling of well-being. One new report says that exposing yourself to outdoor green spaces can even reduce your risk of heart disease, type 2 diabetes, premature death, high blood pressure, and stress.[10] Just looking at nature is good medicine.

And when you can, return the favor. Think about your impact on the environment. Get a little more conscious of how your actions affect your environment and you will see where you can change a few things. Begin by thinking about what you consume and why. Do you choose food that is produced sustainably? Do you use products that add more chemicals to the environment and to your body? You can give yourself permission to decide what to eat and use and do, rather than being unconsciously swayed by advertising or public opinion. You can give yourself permission to take in natural, nutrient-dense food, to make conscious choices about what you put on your skin and what you use to clean your house, to decide to produce less trash, use fewer plastic water bottles, and buy things from companies with values you support, rather than those with values you don't want to support.

How far you take this is completely your choice, but if you don't know and never question, then you might be contributing to a world you don't want in ways you don't have to participate in. We live in a capitalist society, so your choices matter—we all have the power to choose to buy things we know are good for ourselves and good for the environment—because the fate of one is the fate of the other. Brands and businesses change as we change, and your dollars and the energy you spend when you work to earn those dollars can shift the marketplace and begin healing our stressed-out planet.

But permission isn't pressure. Nobody's perfect, and we each do what we can. I certainly have bought things, and probably still do buy things, without an awareness of where they came from. Sometimes it really is hard to know. I am making an effort right now to educate myself more about those things in my life because I'm in a position where I feel able to do that, but maybe you aren't quite ready to take it all in, especially if you are in a state of burnout or poor health at this moment. First things first. You need to find inner balance before you can reach out to work on and support outer balance. Every small thing you do makes a difference, so it's okay to start small. In fact, that small thing can actually have a huge impact if we all make those small choices. Do what you can handle right now. Maybe you start by stepping outside and looking around at nature and just taking it in. Do it for just one minute a day. That is how your brain begins to shift, and the other shifts will happen when you are ready.

EARTHING

Once upon a time in human history, people were in direct physical contact with the earth all the time. We got our food directly from the earth using our bare hands. We walked on the earth—no sidewalks, not even shoes. We spent most of our time outside in the sun or rain, wind or snow. To ancient people, standing barefoot on the ground was just part of ordinary life. For us, it has become so unusual that we have a name for it and consider it a therapy.

The earth has an electromagnetic surface that interacts with your individual energy field. Energy is always moving in and out of the body, and your body is always taking it and giving it. I'll tell you more about how energy moves in the body in chapter 7, but basically we can take in energy through all parts of ourselves, including the tops of our heads and the bottoms of our feet, and we can give energy through our hands (among other places). To keep yourself energized and "charged," you can't just send energy out all the time. You also have to take it in, and the earth is a massive and generous source of energy.

Humans are meant to be in direct contact with the planet for this purpose—there is scientific research showing how *earthing*, sometimes called "grounding," can actually measurably change the body. Earthing has been shown to lower inflammation, improve immunity, speed healing, reduce the symptoms of autoimmune disease, improve sleep quality, reduce pain, improve heart health, thin the blood, and reduce stress and anxiety.[11] Because human flesh is a semiconductor, one theory is that the electromagnetic energy from the earth has an antioxidant effect on the body.[12]

Earthing is as simple as touching the physical earth, but, as you can probably imagine, technology has come into the game. You can buy grounding mats that plug in to grounded electrical outlets that draw energy from the earth. This energy is in the form of electrons that can neutralize free radicals in the body, or so the theory goes.

This is thought by some to reduce stress and inflammation. Grounding mats are often used in research studies that test earthing because they make it easier to control the conditions of the experiment. For example, researchers used grounding mats in a sleep study that showed people who slept on the grounding mats for eight weeks regulated their circadian rhythms and reported less pain and less stress, anxiety, depression, and irritability, compared with people who slept on a mat that wasn't grounded (but looked the same).[13] Another study subjected eight people to a new, intense, weight-lifting exercise that caused leg muscle soreness, then had half the subjects sleep on grounding mats and put grounding patches on their leg muscles and the bottoms of their feet. The other four people used mats and patches that weren't grounded. The grounded subjects experienced significantly less pain, and had more favorable changes in their blood chemistry and inflammation levels, even though they didn't know whether they had the grounded mats and patches or not. They also had steady decreases in white blood cell counts, meaning the body was less inflamed and required less healing intervention, while the ungrounded subjects experienced increasing white blood cell counts.[14]

Earthing is particularly good at reducing stress and increasing feelings of well-being. One study of fifty-eight healthy adults exposed half to earthing through grounded patches on their feet, and gave the other half ungrounded patches. Half the grounded subjects showed almost immediate brain changes, and all grounded subjects showed immediate changes in muscle tension and pulse rate.[15] Another study of twenty-eight people, half women and half men, showed that grounded subjects showed changes that indicated rapid activation of the parasympathetic nervous system (the rest-and-restore system) and a deactivation of the sympathetic nervous system (the fight-or-flight system).[16]

But you don't need a fancy grounding mat to get these benefits. All you have to do, to take advantage of your own conductivity and literally exchange electrons with the planet, is to take off your shoes and step outside. Stand on grass, bare dirt, rock, or sand, or stand in shallow water. Saltwater is even more conductive and is also full of minerals you can soak up through the bottoms of your feet (in case you need another excuse to go to the beach). Standing on concrete in a busy downtown is a totally different experience from standing with your feet in the grass or on the sand or in the ocean. People often say that when they are asked to think of a place that makes them feel peaceful and safe, they think of a place in nature. We all have that instinct that we need nature!

Try it and you will feel it. Give yourself permission to take your shoes off and let your feet rest on the earth. Move your toes into the sand. Sit down on the grass and look at the sky. Lie down under a tree and look up through the branches. Feel the support of the planet beneath you—the earth literally having your back. Close your eyes and focus on how you feel in your body. Most people who practice earthing regularly say they can physically feel the effects.

✦ GROUNDING MATS ✦
AND SHEETS

The most natural way to practice earthing is to make direct contact between your body and the body of the earth, but you probably can't be outside all the time. If you want more frequent contact, you could get an earthing mat to put on your bed or under your feet while you're working. The ones I've seen range from less than $40 for smaller mats to less than $200 for larger mats for your bed. You can also buy grounding sheets. The ones I've seen run somewhere between $35 and a little less than $200, depending on size and style. If you decide to try a grounding mat or sheet, you might want to keep track of any changes in your pain levels and sleep quality. Seeing changes in your physical body and health state can help motivate you to practice earthing more regularly.

GARDENING AND HERBS

Another beautiful way to connect with the earth is to plant things in it, harvest them, and use them yourself. The plants that grow from the earth provide some of the most potent healing foods and medicine available to use, and growing plants can create a powerful connection between you and your natural environment. Growing flowers is a way for you to connect with the earth to create beauty. Growing vegetables and herbs that you eat and use is a way for the earth to literally feed and nourish your physical body. The feeling of taking a vegetable or even a simple basil leaf from your own outdoor garden or indoor plant is a great reminder of how we were once very connected to the earth and its resources and still can be.

No matter where you live, there is almost always a way to grow something. There is a natural and instinctive connection to earth that comes from plants you've grown yourself. When you garden, you are literally putting your hands into the earth, and that earth is going to become part of your body's energy. Gardening gets you outside to pull weeds, thin plants, harvest, and then take in what you've grown. Even a simple indoor herb garden can bring a little piece of the natural world into your kitchen. Taking just a moment to smell your herbs is so rewarding!

In our home, I've planted rosemary and lavender bushes around the house, a lemon tree in the backyard, and the most stunning hydrangeas in the front yard. I do not have a green thumb, but I do know how joyful it makes me feel to smell the herbs as I walk by, to see the flowers, and to admire the lemon tree . . . and the roughly three lemons we get each year!

I love the sensory experience of going outside and picking these fragrant herbs. Other herbs add freshness, flavor, and nutrients to the foods you make at home—you could plant parsley, cilantro, basil, oregano, thyme, tarragon, or chives for cooking, or you could plant tea herbs like lemon balm, jasmine, mint, or chamomile.

But even if you don't grow your own, buying as much food as you can from local growers, such as at a farmers' market or at farm stands, and buying fresh, locally grown produce and herbs from your local grocery, can benefit you in a lot of different ways:[17] Local food that has been recently harvested is fresher, tastes better, and retains more nutrients than food that has to sit in a truck and travel across the country or come from another country. Local food also tends to be available more seasonally, so you can eat according to the natural cycle of the seasons. This is something I try to practice even in Los Angeles, where we don't exactly get the same dramatic seasons as we had in North Dakota. But, for example, I know that peaches are not in season all year long, so I usually don't buy them in winter and instead look for more of the root vegetables and perhaps take in less summer fruit during the winter season. It's fun to look up what's in season in your part of the world throughout the year. Not only are you following the natural cycle and rhythm of your immediate environment, but you'll also support your local economy and small businesses, which can add to your sense of being an active and contributing part of your own community. If farmers' markets are a social event in your town, they also give you the chance to get out and meet your neighbors or just have joyful connection with other like-minded people.

Locally produced food also tends to be safer, with fewer opportunities along the transport chain for contamination, and local growers can give you more direct information about where and how your food was grown. Even just having fresh herbs and fresh flowers in your home can help you feel more connected to and supportive of your health and the health of the earth.

NATURALIZE YOUR INDOOR ENVIRONMENT

The last thing I want to talk about in this chapter is the physical environment you live in. One of the best ways to make a home environment feel positive is to bring more nature energy inside. This can completely transform the feeling you get when you walk into your home at the end of a long day.

Imagine sitting in an all-white room with white plastic walls and no windows, in a white plastic chair at a plastic table. You are sitting under fluorescent lighting and the ceiling above you is made of those industrial, acoustic ceiling tiles. Your feet are on synthetic beige carpeting and there is nothing on the walls and no sound. Think about how you feel sitting in that environment.

Now imagine sitting in a room filled with green plants and potted trees, and a small indoor fountain beside wide-open windows with fresh air coming in. Outside the window you can see trees and a beautiful herb garden—the scent of herbs drifts through the window. You are sitting on a comfortable, beautifully carved wooden chair at a table made out of a thick slab of polished granite with a big bouquet of fresh flowers in the center of the table. Sunlight comes into the room through a skylight and the room is filled with beautiful crystals and chimes. Your feet rest on a warm wooden floor.

How do you feel in each of these environments? You can probably see from this experiment that even in your mind, nature soothes the mind and calms the body. You can't control a lot of things about the world, but you can control many of the things about your home environment. You can make a difference in whether your home environment stresses you out with its synthetic materials and clutter, or if you live somewhere that makes you feel calm and replenished, a place you can't wait to come home to.

To bring the natural world into your home, you don't have to move to the country or completely redo your entire interior. There are many easy ways to increase the positive energy in your home. Some of my favorites are these:

- Crystals and stones placed around the home can help with grounding.
- Large stone and wood elements like granite countertops and wood floors help anchor your home energy so you feel safe and secure in your home.
- Plants growing in pots also bring grounding (and more oxygen) into your home.
- Earth's natural colors, like all shades of brown, orange, red, blue, yellow, and green, evoke earth energy.
- A Himalayan salt lamp is not only a rock, but emits an earthy glow, and may purify your air by infusing it with negative ions, which could boost mood, health, and energy.
- Water contains highly organized energy that can cleanse and purify the body and mind. Bring water into your home with crystal bowls filled with spring water, small fountains, water features, and fish tanks. The sound of water is actually proven to reduce stress—one theory is that each person hears individual noises or "songs" in the white noise of flowing water. This can center the mind in the present moment rather than on distracting thoughts.[18]
- Having natural light and fresh air coming into your home is also refreshing for your physical body.

Another thing I love to do is to light candles or incense, or burn sage or use sound in my home. I usually use these in my rituals, in rooms that feel stagnant, in places where I'm feeling stuck, or wherever the air feels sticky or dense to me. Research shows that when air contains a lot of positive ions, it can cause stress, but that burning herbs can infuse the room with calming negative ions,[19] as well as reduce airborne bacteria by 94 percent.[20]

One study also showed that sage oil can improve mood and memory,[21] and Palo Santo is a traditional remedy for colds, the flu, asthma, and headaches, because of its relaxing properties—and it's also a good insect repellent.[22] Sage is best for diffusing negative energy, so when you want to get rid of a negative feeling, use sage. Palo Santo infuses spaces with positive energy. However, recent media has shown that it is endangered, so I have stopped using it in my home. I use incense when I'm setting an intention, sending up a prayer, or performing any kind of ritual.

For example, after I've had a lot of people over to my home, or if I get a package in the mail and I'm not sure where it's been on its journey, I will sometimes do a quick clearing of the house or the package with sage. I use sage, clearing essential oils, and detox mists or sprays a lot. For instance, I use them when I've been out all day and I feel a heaviness or density when I get home, or if I'm back from a period of stressful travel, a heavy teaching load, or a lot of Reiki work. I may light the sage on the stove and bathe myself in the smoke. I even cleanse my crystals with it. I also use singing bowls and tuning forks to clear stuck or negative energy.

Use these clearing practices anywhere you feel that you need to clean the energy or clear a blockage. Doing this in your home office can free up your creativity and productivity. In the bedroom, these elements can spark passion. In the family living space, they can generate good feelings of togetherness and the warmth of family and friendship.

Candles, fireplaces, and woodstoves bring general fire energy into your home, and are also calming for evening. Firelight doesn't contain stimulating blue light, so it helps your brain to release melatonin for better sleep. Of course, never fall asleep without snuffing your candles!

If weather and allergies permit, open your windows whenever you can. You could also move the air in your home with fans and use wind chimes, mobiles, silk curtains, and anything else that moves with the air to give you the impression that your indoor space has a breeze. Air purifiers can help clean and clarify your indoor air.

FENG SHUI TECHNIQUES FOR
BETTER ENERGY FLOW

Feng shui is the Chinese art of arranging a living or working space for the best possible energy flow. As with Reiki and
other energy-healing practices, feng shui's aim is to maximize
health, vitality, energy, abundance, love, and peace—in this
case, of the environment and, by extension, of the people in
the environment. There is a lot to feng shui and you may enjoy
reading about it and learning more about it, but here are some
basics to spark your interest, which you can try in your own
home:

- Use natural materials whenever possible. They are the best
  conductors and facilitators of energy flow—this includes
  earth, plant, fire, water, and air elements. Plants, pets,
  wind chimes, water features, mirrors, crystals, lights, and
  candles are all good feng shui.
- Arrange your furniture so that energy can flow freely
  around and through it. Don't block doors or windows, and
  people should be able to walk around and through all furniture arrangements.
- Don't sleep under beams or other structures over the bed
  that cut across the bed—these can interrupt energy flow
  while you sleep. This is thought to keep you healthier. Also,
  position your bed, if possible, so someone could get in the
  bed from both sides, especially if you want to attract a
  partner or improve your relationship.
- Try to keep the bathroom door closed and the toilet lid
  closed. This keeps abundance energy from flowing out of
  your house and is thought to increase wealth.

- You should be able to see, but not be directly in line with, the door or opening to any room when you are sleeping, sitting at your desk, or cooking at the stove. If you can't see the door from any of these positions and you can't change things around, position a mirror so you can see the door in the mirror.
- Never keep broken things in the house. Let go of them. If a fixture that can't be removed breaks, like an appliance, a light fixture, a doorbell, or a garage door, fix it as soon as possible. A broken cooking appliance could block nourishing energy, a broken tool could block your ability to fix problems in your life, a broken light could block new ideas, a broken doorbell or garage door could block good fortune from entering your life, etc.
- Don't display too many pictures from the past, or of things that are old, because that vibration can keep you stuck in the past. It's great to have pictures that evoke good memories, but also keep pictures around that are more current. For example, my teacher asked me why I had pictures of my kids at ages five and eight, when they are much older now, because that is like showing them that they can't grow up. I have also noticed that in my parents' home, there are mostly pictures around the house of all of us as teenagers, and I often wonder if that holds them back from living in the present. In general, when deciding which pictures to display, ask yourself: Does this energy match my current vibration?
- Keep your home clean and uncluttered so energy can flow and the universe can perceive that you are prepared for new opportunities, rather than sending the message that you already have more than you can handle.

As you continue to refine your own body and earth awareness, here is a meditation you can use. It is a powerful practice for tuning in to your senses, which are your body's direct method for communicating with the external world.

~~~

FIVE SENSES MEDITATION

Each of your senses has its own way of knowing and connecting with the external world. Honor all of them with this simple meditation:

Find a comfortable seated position. Close your eyes and take a few deep breaths until you feel calm and centered. Give yourself permission to totally immerse yourself in your own sensory experience. You will keep your eyes closed until the last part. Because this meditation is best performed with your eyes closed, I recommend listening to the audio version of this book, or recording yourself reading it.

When you feel ready, begin.

First, focus on your ears. Feel where they are on your body. Imagine opening them to become keenly aware. Now listen. What can you hear in your immediate environment? In your mind, name all the things you can hear. The heater or air conditioner? The fan? Cars driving by? People talking in another room or outside? Birds singing? Wind? Rain? Spend three full minutes completely immersed in the sounds around you.

Next, focus on your nose. Feel it there in the center of your face. Imagine turning up the volume on your sense of smell, then focus on anything you can perceive by smell. At first you might not smell anything, but stay with this sense for three minutes. Do you smell new carpet? Dust? Nature aromas from outside? Food? Can you smell the wet smell of water, or cut grass? Can you smell the flowers on the table, or the faint smell of the dog or cat that lives in the house? Even if you think you can't smell anything in particular, just stay focused on the sensation of smell.

Next, focus on your mouth and its shape. Bring your awareness to your teeth and your tongue. What do you taste? Can you taste toothpaste from when you last brushed your teeth? Can you still sense the subtle taste of the last thing you ate? What does your mouth itself taste like? What sensations can you feel on your tongue? Stay with your sense of taste, even if you can't actually taste anything you can name, for three minutes.

Next, focus on your skin. Feel its protection around your body. Open your awareness to the sensation of touch. Feel everything touching your skin. Every piece of clothing, and where it makes contact with you. Can you feel your hair hanging down your neck or back or forehead? Are you wearing any jewelry or a watch you can feel? Feel the ground under you and how it supports you. Can you feel the air on your skin? The moisture in your mouth and eyes? Can you feel your heart beating, or your pulse? Stay finely tuned to every visceral feeling for three minutes.

Finally, slowly open your eyes. Suddenly there is a whole visual world around you! Try to look at it as if you were seeing it for the first time. Notice everything you see—notice the shapes, colors, textures, the words and images. Look around you with wonder at the amazing visual input—there is so much detail and beauty to see! Take it all in for three minutes.

When you are ready, bring your senses back into balance, take a few more slow breaths, then end the meditation. See if you can continue to notice input from all five of your senses as you move through the rest of your day.

Now that you have tuned in to your body, let's move to the next part of the triad, which is mind.

CHAPTER SIX

The Burning Bright Mind

When the mind is most empty / It is most full.
—SUSAN FERRIER, SCOTTISH NOVELIST

EVERYTHING YOU THINK about yourself, your feelings, your emotions, and your experiences comes from your mind. All your imprints live here, and so does most of your anxiety, depression, worry, fear, and grief. Of the three parts of the triad of wholeness, the mind is often (although not always) the part most responsible for chronic stress. A stressor comes from the outside, but stress happens when the mind perceives that event and reacts—and, in the case of chronic stress, reacts, and reacts, and keeps on reacting.

If you feel constantly stressed, anxious, or burned out, your mind is the place to begin your work. As you heal the mind, healing in the body and spirit will follow, but to heal the mind means more than just "thinking positive" or meditating every day (although both are tools you can use). Most people with anxiety or burnout don't just need to be told to have positive thoughts. Positive thoughts alone cannot defuse chronic stress, an anxiety attack, or fear. In some people, meditation can even make things worse in the beginning and may not be the right initial tool.

If you have burnout, chronic stress, or anxiety, what you really need to do is to get super-clear on your daily, weekly, monthly, and yearly stress levels. If you are always oriented toward doing and accomplishing, or if you know or suspect that you have an anxiety disorder, focusing on stress specifically is the most important thing you can do for your mind.

As we explore mind and what we can do to align it with body and spirit, you will see how intimately connected it is with body. When your mind and body are in alignment, you will experience a delicious state of calm, as your mental life syncs into step with your physical being. Rather than constantly reacting to what is happening around you and unintentionally or unconsciously responding to what other people do, this balance will give you the peace of mind to make conscious decisions about your life. It will also help you to design and project your intentions, define your purpose in this life (or just your purpose for the day), and orient your life toward that purpose.

Knowing your purpose is at the heart of mental health. No matter what happens to you, your purpose can be your guiding light, reminding you why you are here and helping you make decisions about what to do and how to think about things. If you can come back to your purpose, you will never stray too far from your path. In this chapter, we're going to work on how to find that purpose for yourself, how to access your intuition, and how to keep your mental space clear, clean, and spacious, so your brightness can shine through.

A healthy mind leads with intention and focused action. It knows when to activate and it knows when to slow down or quiet down for restoration and relaxation. When your mind is healthy, it feels natural to go with the flow of life. A healthy mind is optimistic, has faith, and trusts that what is happening is happening for a reason. A healthy mind knows that thoughts and feelings move in and out of you, undulating through your mind like waves in the sea. If you ride them with a sense of ease and grace, you won't be dragged down with the effort of trying to keep the ocean still.

But a mind that is anxious, burned out, worried, fearful, or depressed operates without intention, guided by imprints and reactions. A healthy mind acts but a stressed mind reacts. When a mind is out of balance, it will be more likely to fight and struggle against things it can't control. It can lose sight of priorities and goals. Thoughts spiral and perceptions become unrealistic, such as believing that a low point will last forever or that the mind can force a moment of joy to last forever.

You will never get rid of every negative thought, and you don't need to try. Negative thoughts are part of life and of a normal mind. However, what you can do is shift how you attach to your thoughts. You can let them carry you away, or you can observe them as they come and go. You can also curate the content of your thoughts. Just as good physical health means you don't fill up your body with junk food, good mental health means you don't fill up your mind with junk thoughts. You can always infuse your mind with more of the thoughts that make you feel bright. When you let go of your efforts to control the mind and instead work with what is there and in its natural rhythm and time, you will be able to find those calm spots, even during the storms.

But this takes some practice, so, in this chapter, I want to share with you some powerful ways of rethinking, and some things you can do that can help you acknowledge what is happening in your mind so you can learn how to flow with it and color it however you choose. The mind is vast and there is a lot going on in there. Exploring it is an exciting road to understanding yourself.

What Do You Think About?

Have you ever thought about what you think about? The thoughts that flow in and out of your mind are often a response to your environment—figuring out a problem, planning what to do or say, or reacting to anything from your own reflection in the mirror to that thing your friend said to you that seemed kind of mean and now you can't stop thinking about it. You think about what you see, about other people, the next moment, how you feel, what you want. You think about what happened in the past, you think about what's going to happen in the future, and you think about whether you are thinking about something the right way or the wrong way.

Humans think *a lot*. According to an often-quoted National Science Foundation report, the average person has between 12,000 and 60,000 thoughts per day (some say we have even more). And of these thoughts, 80 percent are supposedly negative thoughts, and 95 percent are repetitive thoughts.[1] Think about that for a second. Not only are 80 percent of your thoughts potentially negative, but you aren't even creating enough space and activity in your mind to create *new* negative thoughts! How boring we all are, to spend so much time on negative thoughts that are already used up and worn out and just repeating on a loop!

What are the repetitive thoughts in your mind right now? Really tune in right now to those repeating thoughts. You're probably not even aware that you're thinking them. When you don't bring awareness to the content of your thoughts, negative thoughts can command more of your attention than they deserve. Just because you have a thought doesn't mean you need to latch on to it and have it over and over again. And a negative thought doesn't mean anything about you as a person, or you as the person you're here to be. You can have a negative thought and be aware of it, and then you can let it go so you can put a brighter thought in its place.

But thoughts can be very persuasive. If you look at yourself in the mirror, your thoughts might tell you that there's something wrong with the way you look. You might follow that thought, obsess about it, put it on repeat, until you start to mistake the thought for a truth. Thoughts often come from imprints, but they are not facts. They are just games of the mind—something human brains do. The problem starts when you stop questioning your thoughts and just allow them to keep going with no supervision until they establish their own false reality. You start to believe them, instead of being objective about them, and those beliefs can end up making you unhappy.

Beliefs are just thoughts you've decided to keep, or to label yourself with, or to use to justify what you do and don't do in life. Sometimes that's a good thing, if your thoughts are positive, loving, supportive, and helping. These thoughts can turn into beliefs that bring you joy and are in the service of your highest good and the highest good of others. But when your thoughts are negative, critical, undermining, or self-destructive, they can translate into beliefs that cause you pain for no good reason. You don't have to hold on to those thoughts, those imprints, or those beliefs. You can choose to let them all go. You can choose to surrender your hold on them so, just like strong feelings, they can pass through you and be gone.

Tricks of the Mind

Oh, my love, sometimes the mind can pull us in such directions, it's almost unreal—like when it convinces us that people are bigger than they really are, or that we are smaller. Sometimes the mind will make someone else so big in your thoughts that you feel as if you shrink when you are around them. This could be someone you admire or even idolize. If you have ever been starstruck by a famous person, you have an idea of what this feels like. They seem larger than life! But this can also happen with mentors, parents, highly successful friends, siblings, or teachers. I will never forget a few students who came to me in the past and told me that they stopped following me and coming to my classes because they said that when they were around me, they felt that there wasn't enough space left for them to become the teachers or healers they wanted to become. This was hard for me to hear because it was the opposite of my intention as a teacher. My beautiful reader, if you could see me in person, you would see that I have zero intention of ever making anyone feel small or "not enough," but everyone's mind plays its own tricks and has its own imprints, so I respected that these students needed to move on for their own reasons.

Sometimes the person who seems so large is someone who has hurt you in the past, or maybe someone you hurt. Or it might be someone with whom you have had a stressful interaction and you fear seeing them again. You make them so big in your mind that your mind races at the mere possibility of running into them. Logically, you know this person is just another person like you, but it doesn't feel that way in your mind. If you just bring some awareness to the feeling, you may be able to unhook yourself from that feeling of anxiety.

And if you do encounter that person, remind yourself that who that person is has nothing to do with who you are, and however the interaction goes, that is how it was meant to go and there will be some lesson in it. Maybe it will be much easier than you think, and maybe it won't be, but you don't know right now how it will happen. If you surrender to it and stop trying to mentally control it, you can release the anxiety and let the interaction, if it should happen, simply be what it is without the mind magnifying the person or the occurrence out of proportion. And you know what they say—haters gonna hate and lovers gonna love. What you can give yourself permission to do is let go and love despite what others may do.

Here is another trick of the mind I often see. Sometimes the mind can convince us that the needs of others are more important than our own needs, and this can lead to burnout. One group of people who seem to be most susceptible to burnout are people in the service fields. I have worked with hundreds of people who are out there in the world devoting their lives to the service of others—functional medicine doctors, acupuncturists, yoga instructors, traditional medicine doctors, meditation teachers, nutritionists, nurses, health coaches, healers, schoolteachers, incredible parents, and people with businesses oriented toward helping others. Too many of them are burned out and stressed out in a way that creates negative physical impacts on them and lessens their ability to make an impact on the world, even though that is their passion.

You would think that people who serve others would know how important it is to get enough sleep, nourishment, and periods of calm and relief, but many of them put their own needs at the very bottom of the list. Healers and doctors and teachers often become zapped, and the primary driver of burnout in these people is that they are giving to everyone but themselves. If you are a healer or if your passion is service, be especially aware of your susceptibility to burnout and don't let your mind trick you into thinking that anyone else's care needs are more important than your own. Get some sleep. Eat something healthy. Take a break. The more you fill yourself up, the more you will have to pass along to others. You cannot pour from an empty cup.

~~~~

MIND OVER MATTER

In energy medicine, negative thoughts that stay in the body are thought to result in a density that can actually be a cause of physical disease. If the statistics are true and 80 percent of your thoughts really are negative, that's a lot of density and potential disease, or dis-ease (the body not being at ease). But thoughts can also do the opposite. Positive thoughts have healing power. I recently watched a documentary called *Heal*. In it, Michael Beckwith, a minister and author, said: "Tonic thoughts create tonic chemicals. Toxic thoughts create toxic chemicals."

In that same documentary, there is a story about a doctor named Joe Dispenza who was competing in a triathlon in 1986. During the biking part of the race, he was hit by a truck and was thrown off his bicycle, which compressed six of his spinal vertebrae and paralyzed him. Doctors told him that he needed radical surgery, but even though he admits this is what he would probably recommend for his own patients, he decided against it for himself. He kept thinking, "The power that made the body heals the body." He decided to trust this higher intelligence that designed the body, and offer up his own design for healing. After that, he would step back so that the greater mind could heal him. He vowed to block all negative thoughts from his awareness, then began mentally reconstructing his spine, vertebra by vertebra.

This doctor had a very hard time blocking the negative thoughts, even though he knew the power of positive thinking. He kept thinking of himself being paralyzed for life. But the longer he practiced, the better he got at keeping his mind totally focused on his visualization of his spinal reconstruction. After six weeks, he was able to reconstruct his entire spine in his mind, without getting distracted, and that was when he began to notice physical changes. He started to regain his motor function, was walking after ten weeks, and was training on his bike again in twelve weeks. He had made a vow that, if he was able to walk again, he would devote his life to studying the mind-body connection, and that's what he has done.

What this doctor did, essentially, was learn how to meditate. His focus was the reconstruction of his spine (rather than a mantra or the breath), but as with any meditation, he had to practice to maintain his focus. With steady practice every day, he trained his mind to stay with his intention, and that was when his physical body actually began to change. The spiritual part is that he believed a higher power would heal him, and he was indeed healed, perhaps because he believed. (See page 162 for more information on how to meditate.)

~~~

THE PLACEBO EFFECT AND THE NOCEBO EFFECT: THOUGHTS AT WORK

If you believe something is going to help you, then it might help you based purely on the thought that it will work. This is the placebo effect. And if you believe something will not help you, then it might not help you based purely on the thought that it won't work. This is the nocebo effect. In research, there is always a group testing the intervention (like a new drug) and a control group that is given a placebo— everyone gets the same pill, or whatever it is, but the control group gets dummy pills that don't actually have the medicine in them. Yet, there is almost always a percentage of the control group that gets the results the medicine is supposed to give people, even though they are taking the placebo.

When there is a study of a new medicine that is intended to relieve arthritis pain (for example), some of the people taking the new medicine will experience pain relief (say, 75 percent), but a certain percentage of the people taking the sugar pill will also experience pain relief. The percentage might be lower, but it could sometimes be pretty high—it might be only 30 percent, but it could be 50 percent, or even higher.

Scientists have studied the power of the placebo effect. The placebo effect is most powerful on symptoms that have a thought component, like the perception of pain. But some people think that belief can even shrink tumors and, as in the story about Joe Dispenza and his bike accident, repair actual structures in the body. Studies have demonstrated the placebo effect for pain relievers, antidepressants, anxiety medicine, cough medicine, erectile dysfunction, Parkinson's disease, and epilepsy.[2] The placebo effect is especially significant for drugs prescribed for generalized anxiety disorder and panic disorder,[3] so much so that this effect has interfered with solid evidence of drug effectiveness.

Also, I think it's amazing that up to 85 percent of the reduction of a cough is thought to be related to the placebo effect, with only 15 percent attributed to the actual ingredients in cough medicine.[4] The placebo effect is also strong in cases of irritable bowel syndrome (IBS), which is often associated with anxiety, even though it has very real physical gastrointestinal symptoms. An analysis of the research showed that the placebo response for IBS drugs was responsible for up to 71.4 percent of the drug's effects.[5]

To me, this information is just more proof that the mind is a powerful healer and that thoughts directed toward a specific purpose have more influence than we think on changing our lives. One study showed that even when IBS patients *knew* they were taking a placebo, their symptoms improved anyway![6]

MENTAL HYGIENE

Mental hygiene is the purposeful practice of cultivating positive, productive thoughts in the mind, and it begins the moment your day begins. Just as you brush your teeth and likely wash your face to start the day, mental hygiene is a practice of cleaning and refreshing your mental space before you go out into the world.

Are you aware of what your mind automatically starts to think once you are awake? What are the first thoughts you are conscious of once you've opened your eyes? What do you do first thing in the morning? What thoughts, if any, do you consciously put in your brain when you wake up?

THE COST OF MULTITASKING

According to the American Psychological Association, doing more than one thing at a time, especially when the tasks are complex, costs us all, no matter how good we think we are at multitasking.[7] Multiple studies show that when people do a task repeatedly, such as solving a set of math problems, they can move from one set to the next faster when sticking with one kind of task, rather than toggling between different tasks. That might not sound like a big deal, but if you are constantly switching gears, instead of finishing each task individually, those lost seconds can add up to days, weeks, years over the course of a lifetime—your tasks could end up taking up to 40 percent longer.

Even if you aren't worried about time, a Stanford University study showed that people who multitask the most—what the study called "heavy multitaskers"—are actually worse than people who don't multitask at separating relevant and irrelevant information. They are also slower at switching from one task to another, and had less efficient brain activity, even when they weren't multitasking, suggesting that chronic multitasking has damaging effects on cognition.[8] That alone makes it worth shifting toward more purposefully doing just one thing at a time. It may feel slower, but it's actually faster and healthier for your brain.

One way to start is by setting a timer for yourself when you're working on a project. If you know you have a few things to do in a day, start by time-blocking your tasks and commit to honoring those time blocks. If you need to turn your phone on airplane mode to complete something, do it. While writing this book, I set an alarm for thirty to forty-five minutes and would write and then take a fifteen-minute break so I could refresh and nourish myself or go outside. No matter how much it feels like you have to do, you never need to push the mind or overstimulate yourself in order to complete tasks. It's coun- terproductive. When the allotted time is up, get up and honor the commitment you made so your mind can start to learn how to let go.

You could also make a short list of activities for the day so you can allow yourself to do each item and cross it off as the day goes on. Include some joyful things on the list so you're not trying to do all the more tedious things at once. When you're done working for the day, try making a short list of the things you want to complete the next morning so you can release them from your mind as you shut down your "do" mode for the day. These little active steps of focused doing can help your mind concentrate and give its full attention and ability to a task, so it's done in a more efficient and intelligent way without depleting and stressing your mind's energy.

If you grab your phone before you are even out of bed and start checking social media and answering work emails or text messages, that is what you are filling your brain with, and it will set the tone for your day. Other people's thoughts, other people's opinions, other people's requests will flood your mind before you even have a chance to think about yourself, what you need, and the possibilities for your day ahead.

You don't have to begin your day this way. To practice good mental hygiene, begin your day with practices that fill your mind with calm, peaceful, self-nurturing thoughts before you give your mind's attention to anyone else. Wake up slowly, feeling your body lift out of sleep and into wakefulness. Ease out of bed and do some gentle stretches or yoga poses. Perhaps you stay in bed and do a ten-minute morning meditation or gratitude practice to start the day. Drink a glass of water. Maybe you would like to write down any dreams you remember, or do some free-form writing to open up to the day, or just step outside into the sun for a few minutes. Brew a cup of tea or coffee, relax, and spend some time—it doesn't have to be a long time—contemplating your intentions and desires or purpose for the day. (If you have children, this can be more challenging, but see if you can take time in the in-between moments to do a practice for yourself, whenever you can get it.)

You probably have your list of things you have to get done, but in what spirit would you like to do those things? Do you want to experience your day with compassion? Joy? A sense of playfulness? With ease and grace? Cheerfulness? Do you want to have a quiet day, a high-energy day? Put your intention into your mind before you put it in anything else. See if you can wait until you have showered and dressed and gotten ready for the day before you even look at your phone. If you have to check something on your phone, give yourself permission to only look at that one item and then put it back down again so you can create a sacred morning space for yourself.

At first this might seem impossible. Habits can be powerful, and social media addiction, family responsibilities, and workaholism can fuel that feeling that you absolutely have to get onto your phone or your computer right away. But when you commit your morning to mental hygiene, your entire day can feel different—what an opportunity for you! When you realize how much better this feels and how much more efficiently your mind works if you give it spaciousness every morning, rather than crowding it with external input before your feet touch the floor, you'll recognize why mental hygiene is so valuable and relevant for accomplishing everything you want to do.

You have another chance to practice meaningful mental hygiene before you go to sleep. If you look at your phone, TV, or computer right up until you decide to go to sleep, you are taking all that chaos and external input into your bed and into your dream state. Create a sacred space for yourself at the end of the day, too—it will improve your sleep. Even at midday, you could take a moment to make space for mental ease, peace, reconnecting, and rekindling that relationship with yourself. Every show you watch, book you read, website you visit, or app you participate in has the potential to trigger your imprints, create or reengage old belief systems, and raise or lower the internal vibration of your own energy, so be mindful of your mind and where you put it.

Personal and environmental hygiene can also contribute to a confused or a clear mind state. Sometimes all you need to do to bring peace and calm to your thoughts is to take a relaxed bath or shower—washing your hair, taking time to nourish and moisturize your skin—trim your nails, floss your teeth. Personal hygiene performed like a meditation results in a calm, centered mind and an awareness that you are offering love to your body.

And what about your workday? The state of your desk or work environment can reflect the state of your mind. If you are feeling stressed, feeling chaotic, or having trouble focusing, try cleaning off and organizing your desk or spending ten minutes picking up clutter, if that feels useful. After cleaning up, you can light an incense stick or candle, or place a new crystal on your desk to bring fresh energy into the space. When you start to work again, you might feel more focused or have a new sense of clarity.

Simple changes to your physical space can create big changes in your mind. And simple changes in your mind can create big changes to your physical space as well. When the energy in your home and workspace moves freely, that can calm and clear your mind. Any of the techniques to naturalize your home environment, presented in the last chapter, can also apply to your working environment, as can the feng shui principles I describe beginning on page 136.

But, on the other side, if your desk or workspace or even your home is cluttered at the moment and you don't have the energy to do something about it, or you just know you're not taking a shower today, that's okay, too. The clutter is temporary and you'll shower when you're good and ready. It's where you are at this moment and you can accept that and love on it and let it be what it is. Then, when you're ready, maybe you start with something small—organize one drawer, or let your intuition guide you toward what to do first. Or maybe the right thing to do is to call in a friend to help you get unstuck, or even call in a professional. I've had to have a professional organizer come in to help me straighten up my home when I was feeling too overwhelmed to do it myself.

When the time is right, you will address it. What matters most for mental hygiene is to cleanse and brighten your thoughts and accept where you are right now. You are right on time. Everything is as it should be, and there is something for you to take from every experience. Any practice or action that will put your mind in that place is the right tool for the job, and anything that seems too overwhelming isn't the right thing for you to do at that moment in time. Feel for that spark that says, "Do this!" Let your intuition guide you to what your mind needs most for your highest and best self, and don't be afraid if sometimes it's not to do anything at all.

CHECK-IN TIME:

Let's take a moment so that you can pause and check in with
yourself. Take some deep breaths and focus inward. How are
you feeling? Don't judge, just notice.

HOW WILL YOU SPEND YOUR SUMMER VACATION?

Theoretically, vacations are supposed to give your brain a break so that you can relax and recharge before going back to work. Does that sound like your vacation, or are you more likely to go on family visits that bring up all your old patterns, or party with your friends in Las Vegas, drinking and gambling and staying up all night? Reunions, weddings, birthdays, and holidays can also look like vacations, but be stressful and often, after they are over, cause a big letdown, exhaustion, even depression.

I once did a weeklong yoga and Reiki retreat with twenty-five amazing women in an exotic and gorgeous location. When I got home, all of a sudden my energy dropped and I felt super-low and somewhat depressed. I wanted so badly to feel energized and to get through the day, but I felt as if I could hardly open my eyes or look at my emails. It was really bothering me that I was so tired and almost completely incapable of doing any work for a few days. A teacher of mine had to remind me on a call that week that we are mirrors of the natural world, with its cycles and rhythms and its waves with peaks and troughs (as we discussed in chapter 3). I had been on the peak of a huge wave, where the energetic vibration was very high energy, but eventually when the wave crashed, as they do, I found myself in a place as low as the wave was high. It was actually a gorgeous reminder that it's okay to rest and take it slow after such an active, expansive, and engaged sensory experience with other human beings. It's a permission granter to recalibrate after a big, epic life experience.

If you have been extra busy, working on a big project or operating under a lot of stress, a vacation can give you space to come off all that, even if you don't leave your home. When I've just completed a big project, sometimes I'll do a staycation in a hotel in my town for a couple of nights. Or I might just be off my phone for long stretches of time during the day so I can focus on replenishing myself and not stay so engaged with the things that pull me outside of myself. How can you give yourself space for your mind to relax and release itself from the work it's been doing?

Maybe you could find a retreat to go on that focuses on yoga, meditation, or any other kind of gentle self-care. Maybe a solo trip to a day spa or a rest-and-restore mini-vacation would replenish you, but you don't have to do anything expensive. You could stay home and catch up on your sleep, watch movies, lounge around the house, take your time cooking simple healthy food, take a bath, get a massage, or just hang out with the people you love (or with nobody at all). Whatever spaciousness you choose can give you what you need to build your energy back up again.

YOUR PURPOSE IS
YOUR GUIDING LIGHT

One of the great powers of the mind is the ability to organize and plan actions. This is as simple as thinking about what to have for lunch and as complex as figuring out your purpose on this planet. Your life purpose—or your purpose for your year, or your month, or just your day—is the touchstone for the mind. Do you know yours? Do you have a clear purpose for your life or are you still wondering what it might be?

Some people just seem to know why they are here and exactly what they are meant to do, but most of us struggle with this throughout life. There is no fixed answer. Your purpose in your twenties might be completely different from your purpose in your forties, but if you know your purpose right now, for this stage in your life—or even for this week or this one day—it provides a foundation for your everyday existence that you can sink into and remember when you feel lost or insecure.

Some of my students tell me how worried they are that maybe they don't have a purpose here. This is never the truth. Everyone has a purpose, and your purpose is something that is innate to you. You never have to go outside of yourself to find it. It is something that you have had with you since the day you were born. I often remind my students that right where you are right now, no matter how much or how little you feel connected to your purpose, you are in it and living it and experiencing it in this exact moment. You are already moving in that direction, even if your mind doesn't consciously perceive this. It's all part of your journey to get you to your path and align you with your existence in your current self here on earth.

But maybe you still don't have a clear, conscious idea of what that purpose is ... *and you want to know what it is.* If you aren't sure what your purpose is, start small. You don't play a piano concerto at your first lesson. You start with some scales. So what is your purpose *today*? What do you want to do or be today that will bring you a sense of feeling whole or heart-centered? Could you just focus on something that gives you joy for this one day and let that be enough, knowing that your purpose is within you and it will rise up into your consciousness when you are ready to live it? This is a way to start bringing awareness to the idea of purpose. With each day and each small purpose you choose with intention, your life purpose will gradually come into focus.

But you can also do some work to help you define it and orient with it. One way to do this is to start defining your core values. Your purpose is always related to your core values, so figuring out what those are can help you start to see your purpose forming in your mind. Both your core values and your purpose can guide you throughout your life so that no matter what happens to you in your life, you will have a way to help yourself decide what to do and how to handle the situation. You can always ask yourself if what you are doing right now is in the service of your purpose. Is what you are saying consistent with your core values? If you're being asked a question and deciding to say yes or no, check in with your purpose, even if it is your purpose or intention for that particular day only, and see if it feels aligned with what you want. No pressure, but if you think about this purpose, with its underlying core values, as your guide, then you will always know which way you are going, even if you aren't sure of your exact destination. To help you more clearly define your core values so you can clarify your purpose, see the exercise on pages 176–178.

~~~

JOURNALING

Journaling is one of the most basic and easiest ways to pluck thoughts out of your mind and put them down on a piece of paper outside of your mind so you can become aware of and a witness to your thoughts. Journaling is like catching a butterfly out of the air and examining it under a microscope (then letting it go again) so you can understand what it's really made of.

Not everybody likes journaling, but, for me, it is an exercise of necessity for self-connection. When I write in my journal, it helps me get familiar with what's going on under the surface of my words and thoughts—the programming, the imprints, the subconscious that's running me rises up to the page. When I journal regularly, I get more familiar with what's going on with me, what's controlling me that I might not be aware of, and it's also a way for me to decompress. I might recognize that I'm angry at someone, or worrying about how a situation is going to turn out, or having trouble solving a problem, or trying to control something or wanting something so badly that hasn't manifested yet. Writing about it brings these feelings to the surface so I can process them and see what's really coming up for me. Most of the time it has nothing to do with what I think it's about when I start writing. Recognizing this is a powerful boost to self-awareness.

When I journal, I basically just write freely without thinking about it or planning it, or worrying that it sounds good. In the beginning, I did worry. I made it sort of pretty and in a nice journal and definitely self-regulated in case anyone ever did find it or read it. I remember when I was younger that my little brother and cousin had gotten into my journal and I was so angry at them! When I was older and in my late twenties, my mom told me that she used to go into my room when I was a teenager and read my diary to make sure nothing bad was going on. My journal even had a lock on it! She told me that it was because she was worried about me and wanted to see if I was hiding anything, but I was really upset because it felt like such a violation of privacy. When I started to journal again, I was running on an imprint of mistrust and I sort of policed myself and didn't allow myself the full vulnerability to feel my feelings and write my true thoughts. I wrote as if others might read it.

But now, as an adult and knowing how necessary and important it is to self-connect and journal, I feel safe that nobody will ever read it. I might not even reread it—half the time, I probably couldn't read my own scribbles anyway. It's the process of writing freely more than the content that generates the unfiltered communication with my inner self.

When I journal, I also sometimes write about things that happen in my life—what I do, where I go, whom I interact with, my health progress, where I've traveled to, what I'm working on, and anything else I need to get out of my mind and onto the more neutral territory of the page. But I really love writing out the things that are nagging at me, or about the pain that I'm experiencing, perhaps in my physical body or in my mind, like when I have anxiety or a feeling I just can't shake off. If I'm experiencing something during the day, I might journal when I get home before a dinner out socializing or an evening with my husband so I can get clear and recognize what I may need for myself that evening. Doing journaling or free-form writing before bed also helps me to get troubling, repetitive, or unclear thoughts out of my head so I can release them and sleep better. I haven't forgotten them. I haven't erased them. They may still be there the next day or in a month, but I've given myself permission to see them and put them out there. Most of the time, they change to some degree just through journaling. They don't take up so much of my attention and I can receive rest and surrender, especially before bed.

All you need to start journaling is paper and a pen. You could use an actual journal, a piece of paper, or a legal notepad, anything. Whenever you have the time and feel like taking some space for yourself, just start writing. You might be amazed at what comes up—you might be trying to fix a particular situation, but writing about it will help you realize there is a deeper issue running behind the core problem. Or the solution might just come out of the end of your pen.

You can write freely, or write with a structure. You could ask yourself a question, and then just start journaling freely to answer it. It can be as simple as "How am I feeling today?" or as complex as "Does it feel like I can keep growing if I stay in my current job or am I ready to take this new one?" or "Can I be happy in this relationship?" The answer may not come up right away, but you might get some new insight. You can also journal out any strong feelings—nervousness, excitement, stress. Write through it. You might start with "Oh, I'm so nervous, I'm so scared," but keep going and you can find out why and perhaps even ease the fear and realize that you're just excited about something new. You could clarify an intense feeling, or discover that there's an imprint under there—some old program is running and making you feel uncomfortable about something that begins to feel exciting and fun once you realize you have nothing real to be afraid of.

There's a great quote often attributed to the author E. M. Forster (who may or may not have actually said it, but the quote is great anyway): "How do I know what I think unless I see what I say?" This is the purpose of journaling.

Some journaling prompts and exercises start on page 180.

MEDITATION

Meditation is one of those practices that many people say can only be done one way, but they all have different opinions about what that way is. I believe that there are many ways to meditate and they are all valid. You can study Transcendental Meditation (TM) with a master and sit in meditation for twenty minutes twice a day, or you can lie on your bed and meditate with an app on your phone. You can repeat a mantra out loud or in your head. You can count your breaths. You can pray. You can get quiet and notice every sensation around you to become totally present. You can try to clear your mind and allow thoughts to be like clouds just passing by, or you can let your thoughts go crazy and step back to watch them. You can picture a peaceful environment or your favorite place and imagine that you are there. You can have a teacher guide you through a visualization, a deep relaxation, even a past-life regression. You can learn the meditation techniques of Zen, yoga, loving-kindness, mindfulness, gratitude, bhakti, mantra, or kundalini. You can meditate while lying down, sitting up, observing nature, walking the dog, baking, or running a 5K. Writing in your journal can be a form of meditation. Drinking tea can be a meditation. There are many different levels and different purposes, and they all lead to greater self-awareness.

Personally, I meditate to gain a sense of presence so I can feel fully awake and alive in my present moment, with the purpose of self-awareness. I seek who I am in the now. Just as exercising trains your body and muscles, meditation trains your mind so you are less subject to the whims of thought and better able to feel the presence of the now. I don't believe it matters what kind of meditation you do. Find a form that speaks to you, but do it regularly. There is something beautiful about consistency in meditation. You might commit to meditating ten minutes every day for thirty days, just to see what happens. The incremental shift a daily meditation causes, even if you only sit and breathe for five or ten minutes, can turn into something monumental over time.

In the morning, I like to turn off my alarm, lie back down for five minutes, place my hands on my heart, and just breathe and express gratitude. Then I'll sit up in bed and either turn on a guided meditation so I can just listen and follow a practice for five to ten minutes, or I'll do some easy breathwork to begin my practice. After about ten minutes of either practice, I'll sit in stillness for five minutes. This is the time during my day when I feel most centered, peaceful, and grounded.

After that, I'll do a little bit of stretching and intuitive movement with my body and finish with reiki-ing my heart and setting some intentions for the day. I'll then ask God to guide my thoughts, words, and actions for the day and (I learned this from *A Course in Miracles*, by Dr. Helen Schucman) to show me where to go, whom to meet, and what to say. Even if I'm running late or snooze a bit after my alarm goes off, I rarely leave my bed in the morning without some form of meditation and gratitude practice to set up my day. It's as important to me, if not more important, than brushing my teeth and washing my face.

~~~~~

MEDITATION BASICS

There are many ways to meditate and countless resources for learning the different methods. There are also many guided meditations and visualizations in this book. However, if you want to know the most basic of methods, here is a place to begin. If you can do this once or twice each day, over time you will notice that you gain more calm in your mind and greater ability to direct your thoughts. Meditation is for the mind what exercise is for the body, so the more regularly you train, the more benefits you will gain:

- Sit comfortably with your back straight, either in a chair with your feet on the floor or on the floor with your legs crossed. Set a timer for ten or fifteen minutes, or you may choose to meditate as long as you feel like doing so. Hold your hands in your lap, fingers touching, or place a hand on each knee, palms up or down. You can close your eyes, or keep them open but soften your gaze so you aren't really looking at anything.

- Begin by following your breath. Feel it moving in and out of you. Don't try to control it. Just feel its flow. Stay here for a few minutes.

- After you feel comfortable following your breath, begin to expand your awareness to your entire body. Notice how you feel. Notice where you feel tight or loose; what hurts, what feels good. Don't try to change or control anything. Just be aware. Stay here for a few minutes. If something itches, it's okay to scratch it. If something is very uncomfortable, it's okay to change positions. There are no rules, other than to stay in awareness.

- Now begin to notice your thoughts. Just as your breath moves in and out of you, just as physical sensations come and go, your thoughts form in your brain, float through your mind, and pass away. You will probably feel the urge to follow some of them, letting them engage your mind. Instead, try to just watch them objectively, as if the thoughts were being thought by someone else. Whenever you do get carried away out of the present moment by a thought, as soon as you notice that this has happened, bring your mind back to the position of observer. Stay here for a few more minutes, feeling your breath, feeling your body, watching your thoughts move.

- When the timer goes off or you feel that you are finished, slowly open your eyes, wiggle your fingers and toes, and stretch your legs. When you are ready, get up and keep this awareness inside you as you move on with your day.

Your mind can do amazing things. It can reason, analyze, discover, and create. Expressing your creativity through music (playing it or listening to it), cooking, painting, gardening, singing, drawing, writing, or dancing is a natural and beautiful way to fill your mind with positive, luminous, creative energy. Some people think they aren't creative, but if you are alive, you have been created, and you have creativity within you.

Open your mind to the idea that you could create—it's just putting your visions out into the world, even if you never show them to anyone. You don't have to be a creative genius to create. You can still paint or write or play the piano or dance—sway or harmonize or describe something beautiful in a poem or drench a canvas in colors or draw your own representations of things with a pencil and paper, in a way only you could do. Even listening to music can infuse your mind with inspiration and hope, as you participate in the creativity of someone else who speaks to you.

Whether you join a drum circle or put on your headphones and listen to Mozart, creativity can rekindle your fire and make you feel joyful. When I need inspiration or I just want to feel happier, I always listen to "Fight Song," which was written by my friend Rachel Platten. People call it the "antidepressant song." Every time I hear those words: "This is my fight song, take back my life song, prove I'm alright song, my power's turned on," I get chills and my mind fills up with the amazing feeling that I am here with purpose and worthy of living my best life. Most of us have songs that uplift us or bring tears to our eyes, and those tears are cleansing and beautiful. They help us release things we've been clinging to, and they can bring us back into a state of joy and gratitude for being alive. Try it! Play a favorite song and just be free to feel it and notice what happens.

EMOTIONAL FREEDOM TECHNIQUE
(EFT), OR TAPPING

EFT is a tool for healing and empowerment, stress relief, pain relief, and emotional processing. It's a marvelous and simple therapeutic technique for adjusting energy flow to heal physical and emotional problems. EFT was developed and systematized by energy psychology practitioner Gary Craig in 1995, based on the theory that experiences, such as trauma, do not directly cause negative emotions and physical symptoms (which often have an emotional basis). Rather, they cause disruptions in the body's energy system, and these disruptions cause the negative emotions and physical symptoms.

For example, if you got lost as a child and it scared you, and now you are afraid to go to new places alone, that fear is caused by the energy disruption that happened when you experienced the trauma of getting lost. Or, the situation might be more mysterious to you. You might have pain in your left knee with no known cause, according to your doctor. The real cause, according to EFT, is a block in your energy. It could have been caused by a physical fall onto your knee, or by something emotional, like a conflict that you aren't addressing, so it is manifesting as knee pain. In many healing practices, each part of the body represents an energy of some kind. For example, the knees can represent moving forward in life or accepting change and forward momentum. You don't have to understand the underlying cause to do EFT. Fix the blockage, and the pain can resolve on its own, whether you understand its origins or not.

That may sound a little bit "out there," and I remember thinking it was unbelievable at first, but a lot of research supports both the psychological and physical benefits of EFT. More than one hundred studies on EFT have demonstrated its psychological benefits, but a recent study also analyzed its physical as well as its emotional impact. The study found that EFT was effective at calming the central nervous system, improving heart-rate variability, normalizing blood pressure, curbing the release of stress hormones, boosting immunity, and reducing feelings of anxiety, depression, posttraumatic stress disorder, cravings, and pain, while also increasing feelings of happiness.[9]

To address the emotional or physical pain, EFT works with the body's energy system. This is the same energy system that Reiki, acupuncture, and other energy therapies use. By tapping with your fingers on the end points of the energy meridians in the body or at points where these energy pathways are close to the surface of the skin, the energy moving along the pathways is stimulated to clear the blockages, and this works on clearing the emotional, mental, or physical pain.

I have used EFT to remove a lot of my anxiety and back pain, and the stress I was holding in my body. I cried a lot and still do when I use EFT. I use it whenever I feel stressed out, overwhelmed, anxious, or too excited, or when I feel out of harmony or dissociated from my body. EFT is a great way to get back into your body and to move through feelings of overwhelm. Sometimes I use EFT in my car or on the way to an event if I'm feeling anxious or nervous, or if I'm running late. I'll use it if I wake up in the morning and feel a little blue or if I feel a false heaviness that it's going to be a bad day. EFT can turn that around. I also use it at night sometimes if I'm feeling anxious before bed or restless and unable to sleep. I'll use it after I have an upsetting conversation with someone who triggers me, so I can let an imprint come up to the surface and help to release it.

The beautiful thing about tapping is that you are releasing rather than repressing. Especially if you are new to energy healing or therapy, EFT can be an amazing way to get in and access some of the places where you're holding pain stories and imprints. But EFT doesn't just have to be for pain and for pain stories. EFT is a great tool to open up to receive more abundance, or to just move and shift through different energies inside you, so you can be more open to receiving.

If you want the help of a practiced professional, you could schedule a session with an EFT specialist to do deep therapy work to address trauma and other serious issues, but you can also do some basic EFT on your own. You could do it before doing any of the other practices in this book, to open you up to the power of the practice.

It's important to note that EFT is not a cure for more serious health conditions and proper medical attention is advisable in those cases. EFT is a great resource to support other treatments for any type of medical conditions you may be working through at any point in time, however.

~~~~~

EFT (TAPPING) BASICS

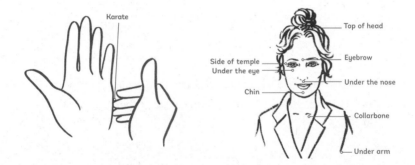

You don't need to see a specialist to do basic EFT on yourself. First, get to know these tapping points and where they are. If you are right-hand dominant, use the following points. If you are left-hand dominant, use the points on the opposite side.

- The outer edge of your left palm.

- The top of your head.

- Right between your eyebrows.

- The side of your right temple.

- Underneath your right eye, on the top of the cheekbone.

- Underneath your nose, just above your upper lip.

- The indentation between the point of your chin and the bottom of your lower lip.

- Your left collarbone, at the inner edge (near your throat).

- Underneath your arm, on the side of your left rib cage.

- The top of your head.

Now that you know the spots, here's how it works:

1. *Decide what problem you want to address. It should be something that is bothering you at the moment—any physical or emotional pain; any sensation like anxiety, a craving, or a compulsion; or any emotion, like fear, pain, anger, grief, panic, or sadness.*

2. *Rate the intensity of the feeling from 0 to 10, with 0 being no problem and 10 being very intense and overwhelming to you at this moment.*

3. *Tap against the side of your left hand with your four right fingers (pointer, middle, ring and pinky) quickly while you say out loud: "Even though I have or am feeling [state your problem], I deeply and completely choose to love and accept myself." Repeat this three to five times.*

4. *Then, repeating the problem (such as "knee pain," "fear of heights," "sugar cravings," "panicking," "anxiety," "overwhelm"), say "I have this [state the problem only]" (such as "I have this knee pain" or "I have this sugar craving"), while tapping on each of the points, in the order listed above, with your dominant*

hand. Do about five taps at each point, then repeat the problem
statement each time you move to a new point. Go in the order
above. You can move as slowly or quickly as you like. As you get
used to the order and memorize it, you can go faster. You can
also start to insert new words or sentences as you tap. To help
visualize this process, I also tell people to find a YouTube video
they feel connected to and utilize that for tapping if they're
just getting started and want a follow-along. There are many
examples online.

5. *Once you've completed a full round of each point, close your*
   eyes and take a couple of deep, releasing, healing breaths. Allow
   the exhale to really support you in releasing. Then with a very
   soft awareness, rate the intensity of the feeling immediately
   after tapping. Has the intensity decreased? In most cases, and
   in most instances, it will.

That's all there is to it. Every time a feeling starts to get intense
and you want to defuse it, just do this (what will become) simple tapping procedure. Sometimes, I do a quick round of tapping for less
than two minutes, and my anxiety decreases significantly. This is a
very effective way to manage the impulse to avoid an uncomfortable
feeling. Tapping helps your body physically process the feeling and
move it out. It might come back, or it might take multiple sessions to
diminish more fully, depending on how deep the blockages are and
how long you have had the pain, but this begins shaking things loose
and letting them out rather than pushing them back down inside.

ASTROLOGY AND HUMAN DESIGN

You might be someone who could take or leave astrology, but I think it's a way to look at imprints and purpose from a celestial standpoint. Even if you have a lot of tools to help yourself and you are doing the work, there are still things happening in the cosmos that could be impacting you and all of us, so why not loop those into your circle of awareness? I choose to believe that where the planets in our solar system were located at the moment of birth has influenced who each of us is today. I think it's so much fun to have my chart done on an annual basis around my birthday, so I can receive some wisdom about the year ahead. I've learned some incredible things and it's made me feel more open and excited about my path as opposed to trying to resist or force something that may be easier and more attainable at different times in my life.

In astrology, you are born under one of the twelve zodiac signs, which is typically referred to as your sun sign. You also have two other very important aspects of your natal chart, which are your rising sign (also called your ascendant) and your moon sign. Once I discovered these other two parts of myself, it made so much more sense to me. Through my moon sign, I learned about my emotional needs, how to heal myself, and how to take care of myself when I'm imbalanced. With my rising sign, I finally understood more about how other people perceive me, which helped me understand how to open up to those parts of myself and then share them with the world in a more authentic way. Rather than fighting what I'm naturally drawn to, learning about these parts of myself helped me lean into them instead. In addition, Chinese astrology, Vedic astrology, numerology, and other mystical systems can help us get to new awareness about our human path and purpose.

For the same reasons, I'm interested in human design, which is a system similar to astrology that looks at planetary imprints and other aspects of the individual. Human design can give you profound insight into your mind, your ways of being, and the innate and intrinsic needs you have as a unique human being, and it also gives you strategies to deal with life in the way that is the most natural for you. In human design, depending on your birth date and time, you could be a generator, a manifesting generator, a manifestor, a reflector, or a projector. These five different designs are all very different (to read more about the complex definitions of these types and discover yours, go to mybodygraph.com). Once you realize which one you are, you will also get to know what your sense of purpose is to some degree and what is most important for you to be balanced and healthy.

To me, the difference between imprints from past experiences and imprints from planetary positions is that one is binding and one is freeing. There were many things my family and society imprinted on me that made me believe I had to be a certain type of person. When I started to learn more about myself, not only through self-awareness, journaling, meditation, and Reiki, but also through things like astrology and human design, I was able to realize that some of these things or traits that I was ashamed of or thought I should change were actually powers that are innate to me.

For example, I have learned that I need to feel free, and I need to follow my own joy. That's not something I can change, and realizing that is who I am on a fundamental level opened me up to a whole new level of self-understanding and self-love. Before, I didn't give myself permission to be that person. I didn't give myself permission to say, "My joy is enough." I often operated in a way that made me want to put others' joy and others' needs of me ahead of my own, which made me feel un-free and disconnected from my own joy. Now I know that my joy *is* enough. I can choose to do something for no other reason than that it gives me joy. I can prioritize my personal joy over my mind's way of making me feel obligated, and I can give myself permission to say yes to things that make me feel free rather than saying yes because I feel bad saying no or because I feel that I don't have a choice.

Understanding where and when you were born naturally connects you to the universe as well as connecting you to becoming who you are in this world. Those attributes are yours, unique to you, incredible allies . . . they are empowering, and there is much to explore. Learn your moon sign to know how to love and nurture yourself as an emotional being. Learn your rising sign so you understand how you present yourself to the world. These can be clues to your superpowers. As I began to explore deeper levels of myself through astrology, that gave me the permission I needed to follow and develop parts of myself that I knew instinctively but not consciously were already in there. It was also a permission granter to myself to start following those intuitive knowings as opposed to trying to make myself someone I thought others needed or wanted me to be. Today those parts of me are some of my strongest, strangest, and best qualities. And, as it turned out, when I started to own them and show them to the world and in my relationships, people began to tell me how much joy it gave them to see me share those parts of myself and how it inspired them to do the same with their own intuition.

You might not be into astrology and that's fine. It's not for everyone. I just want to share with you as many of the practices as I can that have helped me and my clients and students become more authentic to ourselves. Maybe they will help you become more of yourself, and more in love with the you that you came here to be.

As you work with your mind through these many avenues, always remember that thoughts can be useful, helping you to figure out a problem or make a plan. They can help you move toward your goals or fulfill your purpose. But they are only helpers. They don't say anything about who you are or what you are worth or what you will do with your life. Use them as the tools they are—let the negative ones go as you're ready to. Use the useful, pragmatic ones and then let those go, too. Then wait for those new, loving, awareness thoughts that are the jewels that light you up and make you feel so good. Those are the thoughts to follow and lean into. And there are ways to make more of them.

You don't need to feel scared of your thoughts. Give yourself permission to fully and completely embrace the thoughts in your mind right now. That is where your power lies. That is where possibility comes from. If you want to truly burn bright, the thoughts in your mind are the way in. Put your attention on seeing your light, and your thoughts can start to fill you up with that light.

Here are some more mind practices for you to try.

~~~~~

HALT EXERCISE

When you are in a mental state of transition or high feeling, this is not the time to react, respond, agree to something, say no to something, make any major decisions, or discuss something important (especially something emotional) with someone else. The way to tell that it is not time to do any of these things is the HALT test. Ask yourself:

H: Am I hungry?

A: Am I angry?

L: Am I lonely?

T: Am I tired?

If the answer is yes to any of these, put off the decision or the conversation until later and do something to address your physical, mental, and emotional needs in that moment.

YOGA NIDRA

Yoga Nidra is a form of sleep meditation and is one of my favorite go-tos for any afternoon or evening when I am feeling burned out. During Yoga Nidra, you enter into a state between waking and sleeping that is highly restorative and stress-relieving. To do this, I like to take thirty minutes between my workday and the evening to lie down with a gravity blanket (a weighted blanket) over me. I close my eyes and listen to a restorative thirty-minute guided Yoga Nidra meditation recording. If you want to try Yoga Nidra, you can find guided Yoga Nidra recordings on my podcast, *Magik Vibes*. I have them for every season. Lie down, relax, close your eyes, and let the recording work its magic. When I practice Yoga Nidra, I can feel how my whole body shifts. It is one of the most effortless transformations for burnout.

WHAT REALLY MATTERS EXERCISE

I use this exercise to help my students and clients narrow down what is most important to them—their intrinsic or core values—as they are working on defining their purpose for their lives. This exercise helps you get down to what's really important to you at this point in your journey, so you can focus your energy in the direction that is in harmony with where you are at this stage of your life. Here's how to do it:

1. *Get some paper or your journal and a pen.*

2. *Set a timer for three minutes and start making a list, as fast as you can without thinking too much about it, of all the things you think are important to you. They can be big or small, spiritual or material. Anything goes. You might list things like*

family, gratitude, love, success, service, humility, abundance, health, God, or more material or specific things like money, romance, safety, success, children, adventure, beauty, travel, environmentalism, music, animals . . . whatever comes to your mind. Just brainstorm all the things you like and value. If you aren't done at three minutes, you can give yourself one to two more minutes to complete the full list. I'd like you to have about thirty or more words written down.

3. *After you have a list, read it over. It's time to start narrowing down. You will probably recognize right away that some of these things are less important to you than others, but others will be harder, so let's do this one step at a time. Set the timer for two minutes and circle your top ten most valued things on the list. You can start by crossing off everything you know isn't in your top ten, then start narrowing. When you are getting down to the final twelve or fifteen, you may start to have a hard time. To help you, don't think about what you should value. Think about what you actually value. Be honest and remember that this is just how you are thinking today. Tomorrow it could change.*

4. *Now that you have ten things, set the timer for one minute and cross off five items, leaving your top five. My students and clients moan and groan when we get to this level of narrowing down, but the result will be worth it. Really think about which five are the five least important things to you in this moment, and cross them off.*

5. *Now look at those five things left on your list, and cross off three. You can do this!*

6. *Now you are down to just two things—your two top core values, maybe just for today, or maybe in the big picture. Now you know what's next: Circle the one that wins out, even if just by a*

little. Which of these two things is most important to you? This is your core value.

7. *Now that you know your core value, set an intention that today, or for the whole week or even the whole month, this value will be your focus. Set your mind on that word each morning and when you go out into the world, let that word guide you. Write it down and post it somewhere so you see it a few times a day, set a reminder in your phone as an afternoon love note to yourself, whatever you need to remember this is the focus of your mind and your energy today!*

You can always do this exercise again, anytime you want to re-evaluate your core values and priorities and see if they have changed.

~~~~~

FINDING YOUR PURPOSE

If you are feeling lost or unsure of your purpose, whether in the short term or the long term, try this exercise to clarify your goals and passions.

Take a moment to sit comfortably, close your eyes, and relax. Rest and breathe and sink into a feeling of quiet and peace.

Once you feel calm, ask yourself the following questions and answer them in your mind, or write them in your journal, as well as you can in this moment. As you ask each question, take some time to wait. Listen to your heart. See what floats up from the depths of your subconscious being:

- What is that thing you feel deep inside you, that thing you see yourself doing or being that brings you so much joy that it scares your mind to its very core? Don't limit yourself. This can be as wild and big and miraculous as your heart desires.

- What would it look like if you were doing that thing? Just imagine it. Picture who you would be if that were the focus of your life.

- Do you believe you could possibly do that thing, or do you doubt that you could ever achieve it or be that person?

- If you fear that thing, is the fear based in something real, or is it an imprint, or the FEAR acronym: False Evidence Appearing Real?

- What are the things that are standing between your life now and this life you envision for yourself? What are the obstacles?

- What is the difference between you right now and this you that you imagine you could be?

- Look at each perceived obstacle. Is it a real obstacle or is it an obstacle you could overcome in some way at some point, even if you aren't sure how? Do you believe that you can overcome those obstacles?

- Now say these words to yourself: *I am right on time. I am right where I'm meant to be. I am exactly who I'm meant to be. I am going through exactly the things that I need to go through for my highest good. From this moment on, I can go anywhere. I can do anything. I can be anyone. There are no obstacles. Fear is an illusion.* There are no obstacles. *In any moment, there is only me in all my rightness, spaciousness, and infinite potential.* Stay with these thoughts for a few minutes. Breathe into them. Take them into your heart.

- Choose one thing, no matter how small, that could move you one step closer to the life you imagine for yourself. Commit to doing that one thing in the next week or month. Put it in your calendar as a "by when" date. Lean into that reality and keep your awareness in that place.

Release any expectation of result from your action, and surrender it to the universe.

~~~~~

JOURNAL PROMPT:
FREE-FORM WRITING

If you want to get a better idea about what your thoughts consist of right now, one way to see them in black and white is free-form writing. Sit down with your journal, or any piece of paper (a legal yellow notepad is also great) and set a timer for five or ten or twenty minutes. Start writing whatever you are thinking. It doesn't have to make any sense. Don't worry about spelling or grammar, and don't look at what you write with a critical eye. Sometimes I can't even read my words because my writing becomes more like a scribble of thoughts coming out. You can even start by writing "I don't know what to write blah blah blah." Or "What is something I don't want to write about or look at right now?" Just let your thoughts flow from your mind into your heart, like sand in an hourglass, and then down from your heart and through your arms and out your fingers onto the paper.

When the timer goes off, stop writing. Take a few deep breaths, then go back and feel into what you wrote. It will give you an amazing connection to the content of your thoughts. What things were positive? What things were negative? Can you estimate a percentage? Are you hurting somewhere or following an old imprint you weren't aware of?

Knowing what you are thinking is like getting your bloodwork done. If you see something negative, that is good information. Examining your thoughts raises your awareness about your own mind content, so you can consciously choose what to focus on. Free-form writing can show you the random and sometimes ridiculous nature of the thought flow. When you look at those thoughts on paper, you can see that most of those thoughts are not worth much attention. That's not a judgment—remember that what your thoughts are don't reflect what and who you are. Thinking is just something you do, but the more you understand the content of your thoughts, the more you have the power to support yourself in shifting away from junk thoughts to bright thoughts that can bring you peace and ease.

~~~~~

JOURNAL PROMPT: FREE

If the day has gone by and you're feeling disappointed, angered, or annoyed at how much you *haven't* done for yourself, recognize this as a cue for you to tune in to your body and feel where you may be stuck. Where do you feel that your freedom is stifled? To get unstuck, you can do a deep dive into yourself to reestablish your inner sense of freedom. This is a challenge from you to you to access your limitless inner power so you can speak the truth better and love yourself and others more genuinely. In your journal, write the letters F, R, E, E, vertically down the left edge of your page. After each letter, answer the following prompts:

F: FEEL YOUR FEELINGS. Think about your relationships with others. Which ones make you feel hindered or trapped? We are all sensitive beings and sometimes we let relationships get the better of us. Sometimes they are begging to be released and we are holding on too tightly, and sometimes they are just begging for something to change. Try to move inside those anxious, vulnerable feelings about the relationships in your life that aren't working the way you feel they could. Then, make a list of all your relationships under the letter F, and make a check mark next to the ones that make you feel free. Make an X next to the ones in which you do not feel free. You don't have to solve anything. This is only awareness. Just make the list, and make your checks and Xs.

R: RELEASE THE OLD WAYS. You want to break the patterns holding you back from feeling free, beautiful, vibrant, abundant, and your most aligned self, but old habits are hard to break. Under the letter R, make a list of all the bad habits and patterns you want to break but are having trouble releasing. After each item, write something that best describes why you are holding on to that thing you don't really want in your life. It could be something tangible, like "Financial problems: I don't have enough money coming in," or it could be something emotional, like "Obligation: I feel as if I can't get away because they need me." Again, you don't have to solve the problems right now. You are simply elevating your awareness.

E: ENGAGE WITH YOUR HEART, NOT YOUR MIND. Your needs and your truth matter and are your priority. What does your mind think about this statement? What does your heart think about this statement? Under this first E, make two lists: Head and Heart. Under each, make a list of the thoughts or words that come to mind when you tell yourself, "My needs and truths matter and are my priority." What does your head say about this, and what does your heart say about this? Which responses seem the most true? The most useful? The most real to you? The most possible? Reflect on the differences.

E: EXPRESS YOURSELF. Your feelings can teach you about yourself if you fully bring your awareness to them. Under the final E, make a list of all the feelings you remember having felt in the past twenty-four hours. List every feeling you can remember—boredom, amusement, sadness, hope—and what you were doing at that moment that sparked that feeling. Then, without anyone else listening, practice saying each of these things out loud, such as, "Today I was bored when I . . ." or "Today I felt really sad because . . ." Start with the easy ones and work up to the more intense feelings or the feelings caused by more complex situations.

This week, check in with your FREE periodically and keep in mind what came up that was new to you or interesting. These are all clues to begin changing how you show up for yourself and your daily interactions, and to identify what kind of life you really need in order to feel that sense of freedom in which all things become easier.

〜〜〜〜

JOURNAL PROMPT:
WHAT WOULD IT FEEL LIKE?

To help you open your mind to more peace and ease in your life, try this journal prompt:

I wonder what it would feel like to feel _____.

Fill in the blank with any feeling you would like to experience. Do you wonder what it would feel like to feel pure joy? Calm? Free of guilt? Playful? Truly happy? Respected? Fun? Sexy? Brave? Inspiring? Smart? Powerful? Worthy? Whatever word you pick, write about how you think it would feel. Do as many as you feel you want to do, or do one each day for a week. This kind of mental curiosity allows you to begin feeling and exploring the vibrations of your future, soon-to-be life.

JOURNAL PROMPT:
WRITING THROUGH A SHIFT

An exercise I give my students is to write through the experience of shifting in their lives. I give them the first prompt and they write about it, then I give them the shift prompt, and they write about that, and so on. This exercise can be quite revealing. Here are some of the prompts I use. Choose any that seem relevant for whatever shift you are going through in your life:

- PROMPT: What am I most ashamed of about myself?

- *shift prompt:* What am I most proud of about myself?

- PROMPT: What behavior or habit am I fed up with and would like to change?

- *shift prompt:* What behavior or habit have I already changed for the better?

- PROMPT: What am I most anxious about?

- *shift prompt:* What do I feel at ease about?

- PROMPT: Where do I hurt?

- *shift prompt:* Where do I feel healthy?

- PROMPT: Where do I feel scared?

- *shift prompt:* Where do I feel safe?

- PROMPT: Where do I feel weak?

- *shift prompt:* Where do I feel strong?

- PROMPT: What part of my body is storing weakness?

- *shift prompt:* What part of my body is storing my power?

- PROMPT: What situations make me feel small?

- *shift prompt:* What situations make me feel big and bright?

~~~~~~

DREAM JOURNALING

Dreams are the mind's way of cleaning house, and they can reveal subconscious truths about what is on your mind, but because the memory of dreams fades so quickly, it can be enlightening to write them down. Keep a journal and a pen next to your bed so you can write about your dreams before the memories dissipate. To help you remember your dreams, set an intention right before you go to sleep that you will remember them. This might not work at first, or not work in a way that is obvious to your conscious mind, but keep doing it every night for a week and be ready as soon as you wake up to write down what you remember about your dreams. Then, once you've been able to look back and read a few entries, observe any patterns, experiences, and references to notice how they mirror or add illuminating elements to your current life.

CHAPTER SEVEN

The Burning Bright Spirit

Spirituality leaps where science cannot yet follow,
because science must always test and measure, and
much of reality and human experience is immeasurable.

—STARHAWK, AMERICAN WRITER

W E ARE ALL connected by energy, my love, and I am so excited to talk to you about this subject because it's my very favorite part. Energy is the source of all life and connects all life—each of us to each other, to our communities, to our planet, and to the transcendent source of all energy you might call God or Spirit or Universe or Love or Higher Self. Energy runs over the planet like a sparkling, pulsing web of light, through our bodies and in and out of us, between all people and between all things. It binds families together, it connects friends and partners, and it winds between communities and cities and countries and all over the world. Energy moves through nature, between birds, mountains, rivers, clouds, tiny blades of grass and giant mountain ranges, and through everything we have ever made, from buildings and bridges to clothing and computers.

Energy draws people toward one another, which is why people seek out other people and form social groups, why animals seek out other animals and move in packs, flocks, pods, herds. It's why trees grow together in forests and why waves roll in one after the other. Energy moves down deep into the earth to its core, and all the way up, through the atmosphere and into space. It underlies consciousness and animates all beings. The energy of life has its own pulse, and we are all a part of it. It breathes through us, and we give it form. It is magical and mystical and sacred.

✦ CHI, KI, PRANA, ✦
LIFE FORCE ENERGY

Energy is everywhere, and the more you tune in to it, the more you will be able to feel it. Have you ever noticed that certain places just feel good, and certain places feel bad? You can walk into a house or a room and think, "Wow, it feels good in here!" That's your knowingness that it's safe, that you're surrounded by other benevolent beings and by a sense of peace, love, and community. Other places can feel dark, stagnant, stuck. You may even feel that you have to get out of the place immediately. That's your knowingness that it's not safe or that it's not healthy, or that there are other beings around you who are in a bad place. What you know deep inside yourself in that moment is a sense of the energy in those places, as well as the energy emanating from the people around you.

The idea of universal or spiritual energy that flows in and through all things exists in many different spiritual traditions. It may be described in different ways, but we are all perceiving the same thing. This energy can flow freely, but it can also get stuck or stagnant, both in external places like buildings or outdoor locations, and inside your own body. In Chinese medicine, they call this energy *chi*, and this is what acupuncturists manipulate for healing. In Japan, they call it *ki*, and this is what Reiki practitioners manipulate for healing. In yoga and in Ayurvedic medicine, they call it *prana*, and yoga, meditation, and diet facilitate its movement. Later in this chapter, I'll walk you through an exercise that will help you to feel this energy with your own hands.

People used to understand at an instinctive level that we are all part of one great energetic design. People in communities came together naturally to support each other, help each other, and enjoy each other's company. Families stayed together, often in the same house, caring for children and their aging parents and grandparents, from birth to death, sometimes for generations. But ever since machines began to do the jobs humans used to do, forcing people to leave their communities and find other ways to earn a living, people have been moving more and communing less. Now we are in the strange new position of being able to have a conversation with someone on the other side of the planet, and to form groups of people with common interests who live all over the world, all through technology. And yet, people seem to feel more anxious, less supported, and more alone than ever.

We all have a need to connect, not just with a computer keyboard but with physical touch, emotional bonding, and spiritual gathering. It's built into our DNA. Without it, we suffer from energy leaks that manifest in us as loneliness, anger, fear, and sadness. We can even get sick as a result. The energy we get from social connections affects the body—according to an article in *Psychology Today*,[1] scientists have known for decades that the number and strength of social connections influence health more than smoking, high blood pressure, or obesity. More and stronger social connections lead to stronger immune systems, higher self-esteem, more empathy, better cooperation, greater trust, and longer lives.

People who are going through chemotherapy for cancer do better when they have more social support and human interaction,[2] and people who have had a heart attack are over twice as likely to die from a second heart attack if they are socially isolated than if they are socially connected. Having close friends into old age seems to reduce the risk of developing dementia, and, according to one study of people over 80 years old who all reported being psychologically healthy, the people who had more friends and rated their social relationships as the most positive were much more likely to have the memory and other cognitive abilities of people decades younger.[3] Social isolation has been linked in numerous studies to many, many other health problems—not just cancer, heart disease, and dementia, but hardened arteries (atherosclerosis), high blood pressure, slower recovery from illness, and even slower wound healing.[4] Isn't that amazing? If you don't connect with people, your wounds won't heal as fast as they will if you do!

One of the most common reasons people seek out therapists is loneliness, and even back in 1985, Americans claimed to have only an average of three people to confide in (according to a 2006 study published in *American Sociological Review*). By 2004, that dropped to one person, and today, 25 percent of Americans say they have nobody they can confide in (according to a 2019 poll of two thousand Americans commissioned by the counseling service BetterHelp). I did an Instagram story after becoming aware of the loneliness facing so many people. I asked my followers, "Do you feel you have a community you can rely on?" The results astounded me: Forty-five percent of the people who responded said no. Just imagine what those numbers will look like in the future if we don't consciously begin recognizing our need to connect with one another on a deeper level.

There's a theory that language developed because our earliest ancestors needed a more advanced way to communicate in order to work together in social groups for survival, but *survival* has come to mean much more than protection from wild animals or attackers. It's come to mean physical survival, mental survival, and spiritual survival—the survival of all parts of your triad of wholeness. Psychologists through the years have always agreed that connection is a fundamental requirement for humans—we are social beings and we need each other. This is why the most extreme punishment for prisoners is solitary confinement, and why social isolation is used as a form of torture for prisoners of war.[5] According to psychologist Susan Pinker in her 2017 TED Talk, "Social isolation is the public health risk of our time. A third of the population says they have two or fewer people to lean on."[6]

In the *Psychology Today* article I mentioned earlier, the author quoted TED Talk star and best-selling author Brené Brown, who is a research professor in social work. I love what she said: "A deep sense of love and belonging is an irresistible need of all people. We are biologically, cognitively, physically, and spiritually wired to love, to be loved, and to belong. When those needs are not met, we don't function as we were meant to. We break. We fall apart. We numb. We ache. We hurt others. We get sick."

Emma, the twenty-one-year-old daughter of one of my students, is a good example of this. After she graduated from high school, Emma started college but she didn't bond with her roommates, who were all from very small towns. She felt alone in her classes and couldn't seem to make friends. At first, her grades were great, but the lonelier she got, the less she went to class. Every weekend she wanted to come home, making it even harder for her to make friends.

Finally, Emma knew she couldn't keep going, so she decided to take some time off. She moved into a studio apartment by herself—it was a tiny studio with a mattress on the floor. She couldn't afford to have a TV or an internet connection, so she had no connection to the outside world. This made her situation even worse. She became more depressed and anxious, and developed a panic disorder. She stopped paying attention to her personal hygiene and stopped cleaning her apartment. When she met some people in the parking lot one evening, she was so desperate for human contact that she befriended them, but they turned out to be drug users. She began taking drugs, too, because it made her feel less sad and anxious, but of course this just made her situation worse. When the drugs wore off, she felt worse than before, and the friends turned out not to be friends at all, stealing money from her apartment when she was at work.

When Emma's mom found out what was going on, she convinced Emma to go to rehab in Minneapolis. Emma didn't want to go at first, but as soon as she checked in, things began to change. The therapy was useful, but she said the biggest difference was that suddenly she was in the center of a community of people who were all going through what she was going through. She had a roommate. In fact, she was required to be around people all the time—none of the rehab residents were allowed to go to their rooms alone during the day. She fought against this at first, but then the energy of connection began to work its magic on her. She had group meetings every day and social activities every night. She began to feel better, and for the first time in a year, she began to think that maybe she could stop taking those drugs and be happy without them.

After she was finished with her program, she went to AA meetings to continue her connection with people. She moved into a house where she rents a room but has other people around. They often hang out together, watching movies or having dinner. And she got a job at a coffee shop, where she met people she liked and gets to interact with customers all day long.

Recently, Emma told her mom, "When I'm home alone, it hurts, and the first thing I think of is how I wish I could do drugs again. I don't do it, but I think about it. I can be lying on my bed with no energy, binge-watching Netflix, but if someone calls me to go do something or if someone comes over to visit, suddenly I get filled with energy! I want to take a shower and look nice. I want to clean my room. I turn off the TV and the computer and I go for a bike ride or a walk, and I feel so much happier." Emma says she is out of the woods, but she is still standing next to the woods. Every day, though, she inches herself a little bit further away from the woods and toward other people. This is the power of social connection: Without it, people sink. With it, they rise.

In my own work and practices, I've seen firsthand the power of these reconnections to spirit, individually and collectively, during my retreats. One of the reasons these experiences are so powerful for people is that they get out of their day-to-day routines and they try new things with (typically) all new people. By the end, they are crying together, laughing, hugging, and connecting in ways sometimes more powerful than how they ever connect with some of their own family members, best friends, even life partners. They then get to take it home with them and make new choices each day to keep connecting, to keep growing, and to keep showing up for life in its fullest form, with themselves and other human beings.

Dr. Pinker said, "Face-to-face contact releases a whole cascade of neurotransmitters and, like a vaccine, they protect you now, in the present, and well into the future, so simply . . . shaking hands, giving somebody a high five, is enough to release oxytocin, which increases your level of trust, and it lowers your cortisol levels, so it lowers your stress."[7] She also said that social interaction triggers your body to produce dopamine, which kills pain and gives people a little bit of a high, like naturally produced morphine. For fun, I ask people on retreats to try to give and receive a total of twelve hugs each day. It literally lifts people up, and they realize by the end of the retreat how much joy they feel being connected to other humans each day.

CHECK-IN TIME:

Let's take a moment so that you can pause and check in with yourself. Take some deep breaths and focus inward. How are you feeling? Don't judge, just notice.

BLUE ZONES

Around the world, there are certain spots where people live much longer and are much healthier than everywhere else. Journalist Dan Buettner calls these "hot spots of longevity" Blue Zones, and he has written several books about what these people do that are different from what most of us do.[8] The Blue Zones he identified are Ikaria, Greece, which has one of the lowest rates of middle-age mortality in the world, and the lowest rates of dementia; Okinawa, Japan, which has the longest-lived women in the world; the Ogliastra Region, in Sardinia, with the highest concentration of men who have lived to a hundred or longer; Loma Linda, California, where people generally live ten more healthy years than the average American; and the Nicoya Peninsula, in Costa Rica, which has the world's lowest rate of middle-age mortality and the second-highest number of men who have lived to a hundred or older.

You could probably guess some of the things these places have in common, but others surprised me. The people in these communities didn't "work out." None of them exercised at a gym, and none of them went on diets or took any supplements. What they did do, however, are specific things that each fit somewhere into the Burning Bright Triad of Wholeness:

Body: The people in Blue Zones have naturally active lives, so they move a lot. They don't overeat, they tend to eat mostly plant foods, and they eat a small serving of meat only once or twice a week. They also drink wine moderately. (Yay!)

Mind: The people in these small communities all have passions. They have something they live for and love to do—a life purpose beyond their jobs. Several of the Blue Zones have a name for this sense of purpose that translates to "Why I wake up in the morning." They also have different kinds of meditative practices, which can strengthen their ability to bring peace to the mind.

Spirit: This was the big one. Not food, not exercise. The people who live longest in the world all have spiritual practices that feed their souls, bring their community together, and fill them with spiritual energy. Some of them pray, some have ceremonies honoring their ancestors, some just get together and talk about how they can support each other. But most of them are part of a religious community (denomination didn't matter) and attend religious services regularly. Each one of these communities is also filled with close-knit circles of supportive friends and regular social gatherings, formal or informal. And they prioritize family, with committed life partners and a focus on spending time with children, taking care of parents and grandparents, and keeping family physically close, either in the same home or in a neighboring home. For some of us, that is what friends feel like in our lives when family lives far away.

SPIRITUAL CONNECTION IN THE MODERN WORLD

Remember when the seventh day of the week was considered a sacred day of rest? Whether Saturday or Sunday (depending on the religion and how you count your days), nobody was supposed to work. Stores were often closed, nobody could sell alcohol, and people came together with a spiritual purpose and worshipped the higher power of their chosen religion, often standing side by side, singing, chanting, praying in a place dedicated to spiritual practice. Many people followed (and still do follow) these practices with a meal or with breaking bread together in some way.

I remember every Sunday, growing up, we would meet my grandparents at church, and then we would all sit around the church cafeteria with the other families who had attended the service. The adults would drink coffee and chat while the kids ran around drinking juice and begging their parents to let them have two doughnuts instead of just one. Many religious services have a social time after the service, for exactly this reason—to reinforce the community spirit within the religious practice. In many religions, including mine, there were (and still are in some cases) also seriously observed days of fasting, days of worship, and days of commemoration. Rituals were important.

Rituals—at least, sacred ones—have lost much of their meaning, and many people don't go to religious services anymore. Some people still attend church, synagogue, or mosque, but, according to Gallup, the numbers are lower than they have ever been.[9] Between 1937 and 1976, about 70 percent or more of Americans attended religious services regularly. This dropped to about 68 percent by the 1990s, but since the turn of the twenty-first century, there has been a sharp drop-off of almost 20 percentage points, down to around only half.

The number of people who say they have no religious affiliation has risen from 8 percent in the year 2000 to 19 percent today, but even those who do claim an affiliation are much less likely to go to any place of worship than they did in the past. In 1999, 73 percent of US adults who said they had a religious preference belonged to a house of worship. Today, only 64 percent of people who identify with a specific religion attend any services. Part of this trend may have to do with age, since older Americans are much more likely to be members of a congregation. Of people who were born before 1945, 68 percent attend religious services. That drops to 57 percent for baby boomers, 54 percent for generation X, and only 42 percent for millennials.

I was raised as a Catholic and I still feel deeply connected to those Catholic roots. I still love practicing many of the Christian or Catholic traditions that I was taught. It's where I learned to have a relationship with God, and I now feel comfort and safety in that spiritual space because it complements other parts of me and my practices for body, mind, and spirit. Many people have asked me over the years if practicing yoga, meditation, and Reiki is considered sacrilegious, and my answer is quite simple. I believe God wants me and you to be happy and to thrive in this life, and in order for me to feel and emote and move energy and sadness and pain through me, I need more than just praying. I have to work on being whole, and all of these practices help me feel that way.

My mind will go to very controlling and anxious places without meditation. My body had a lot of pain when I first learned about Reiki, which Reiki helped me heal. Movement and breath helped me feel more open, more joyful, and more connected to myself and the world, so I choose to practice yoga, which represents union. For me and for many of my students, these practices are the things that connect us to a healthy and balanced mind, body, and spirit. I don't believe this contradicts any religion. I don't believe there is a one-size-fits-all model for spiritual practice. We are all so incredibly complex and unique! It is up to each individual to explore within themselves what works and fits best, so we can give ourselves the balance and harmony available to us in a very busy, anxious, fast-paced, and technology-based world.

With all we've gained in the modern world, we've forgotten a lot. But we can find it again—maybe not in the same way our ancestors did, or exactly the way they do in the Blue Zones, but we can translate those same ideas to our lives here and now. We can come together in better ways. We can prioritize our relationships with more care. We can reestablish rituals in our lives. And we can re-forge our connection to something greater than ourselves, even if that something is community or nature or a mindfulness practice.

We haven't really lost anything and we aren't really missing anything. It's just that our culture has been changing in a way that overlooks the potential for spiritual health that we all have inside us. To reclaim this potential requires only an awareness of the energy that connects us—the same energy that has always been, and is, and always will be. You can cultivate that energy in your life and receive more profound awareness of the sacred nature of life, your importance in it, and the human connections that can give you ever more spiritual energy for you.

~~~~~

BETTER RELATION-ING

As our energy reaches toward other beings and their energy reaches toward us, relationships inevitably form. We all want to feel that other people care about us and that we are supported. Solid human relationships are good for your health. Without them, you can feel that your life doesn't make any difference, but having relationships comes with its own set of challenges. When you connect to another person or a group of people—the energy web of a family or a group of friends or people who work together—each person's imprints can get activated. You may become too caught up in your own fear of vulnerability, the impulse to control, the compulsion to cling, or anxiety about making a commitment to someone.

We may try to control each other, tell each other what to do, or manipulate the course of the relationship. This can be one of the most difficult challenges of connecting. If you have been working on yourself, you may feel that you should also "work on" the people you care about by telling them how they should handle situations or how they should act or what they should become. This is a very easy way to get caught up in other people's stuff. It also distracts you from your own issues and the ways in which someone else's issues trigger your own, which can make you deeply desire to control or change them, when what you really deeply need to do is let them help you see yourself more clearly.

At one point, I thought that if my husband didn't go down the spiritual path with me, I'd have to get divorced. This was just another attempt at my control—another story of fear that wasn't true. Then a teacher said to me, "Just go do what you want to do for you and let him take his own path at his own time. That's not for you to worry about or control." Huh. I wasn't sure about that, but as soon as I surrendered my perceived control over him, the minute I stopped asking him, "Are you going to meditate today? Do you want to go to yoga today? Will you come do this moon ritual with me?" and just went to yoga on my own, he started asking to come with me. As I write this, he happens to be at yoga right now . . . *by himself!* Sometimes he does more yoga in a week than I do, and now he has his own morning meditation practice. Surrendering my control allowed him to discover that he actually wanted to do the things I wanted for him, too.

It doesn't always work out this way. The people you are trying to control won't always suddenly do everything you want just because you stopped trying to make them do it. But everything we go through leads us a few steps further along our own path. Every challenge, every misconception, every supposed wrong turn, brought you to this place right now. It all prepared your mind and your heart for these truths and this awareness of yourself that you may not have had before. In the end, what anyone else does, or thinks, or sees, is not up to you. The only thing up to you is *you*, and as soon as you recognize that, you can put your energy into awareness of who you are right here and now, and let all the rest go.

You have your own stuff to work out. We all do. You have your own imprints and fears urging you to try to control your situation by controlling others, and people you are in a relationship with have their own imprints and fears that urge them to try to control their situation by controlling you. We all do it sometimes. It's natural to want to fix other people, especially when you think you can see exactly what is wrong with the way they are living, but this is not your job here in this life. You are your responsibility. Your emotions are yours to feel, your body is yours to support and love, your soul and spirit are here with a purpose, and it's not the same purpose as anyone else's purpose. Theirs is for them to work on, and yours is for you to work on. The more you recognize this and begin to loosen your grip on your loved ones, the more your burnout, pain, and anxiety may lessen, and the more easily they will be able to take responsibility for their own needs.

Helping people, being of service—those are productive paths. If someone asks for help or advice, you can reach out to them in kindness and with compassion. You can share the things you've learned from the places you've been during your journey. But controlling, fixing, or giving too much to other people compromises the energy connection between you and them, and will likely leave you feeling depleted, exhausted, and possibly even resentful. And it never really works to try to control someone else, anyway.

To help you better understand the nature of your own relationships and the level at which you may be trying to control them, let's look at these three types of relationships: independent, codependent, and interdependent:

- An **INDEPENDENT** relationship is two people moving along in parallel without any real intimacy in their relationship. Their energy is pretty disconnected because they are both aware of themselves and doing their own thing without really putting any energy into the mutual relationship. Ava is a friend of mine who had a marriage like this. She and her husband were friendly, but they lived more like roommates, rarely doing anything together and never cultivating any real emotional connection. The marriage was civil, but it didn't last because, after a few years, they both felt like they were missing something, and the relationship felt pointless.

- A **CODEPENDENT** relationship is when someone else's needs matter to you more than your own. The energy of this kind of relationship usually runs mostly in one direction, or it is imbalanced. I had this sort of relationship with my mother, who has suffered from depression for most of my life. If she wasn't well, then suddenly I wasn't well and I would start to spiral into my own myriad health problems. She never encouraged this in me, but I don't think she saw it happening, either, because she was too immersed in her own problems. I did it naturally, constantly focusing on her well-being, not recognizing that I made it more important to me than my own well-being.

- What we all seek is **INTERDEPENDENT** relationships. When you are in an interdependent relationship, you know that someone will show up and be there for you when you need it, and you know that when they need it, you'll show up and be there, too. In these relationships, energy flows back and forth freely in both directions. To me, this is the basis of healthy relation-ing—a sense of autonomy of self and an ability to know what you can give and what you cannot give, along with a willingness to share. This creates a relationship between two people who are both in their own truth, but who are also open to trusting and accepting each other just as they are, with genuine love and interest, but without any demands for change or control.

Each of us, including you, has to work on our own inner relationship with ourself first. Each of us has our own inner light, and it wants to burn bright. Each of us has our own path and purpose to follow, and every path is imperfectly perfect, no matter how hard or easy it feels to follow it. To control another person—or to believe you can control their path, their joy, or their pain—is to diminish and ignore the incredible complexity, divinity, and infinity that is within that person.

How do you know what other people's path is meant to be? You don't. And how do other people know what your path is meant to be? They don't. To believe in any way, shape, or form that any of us have the responsibility to manufacture or manipulate the way someone else lives is delusion. Nobody else's happiness is your responsibility, and your happiness is nobody else's responsibility. Nobody else's health is your responsibility, and your health is nobody else's responsibility. Nobody else's joy or pain or needs are your responsibility, and the sooner we can all take ownership of ourselves and meet our own needs as much as possible each day, the sooner we can all get back to experiencing life together, the way we are meant to experience it— with each of us living in our own fullness so we have the energy, compassion, and love that can help to repair the pain and suffering in our world.

When I'm working with a client or on a retreat, I can hold space for someone and support them in opening up to themselves and their needs and feelings, but I cannot do the work for them to keep showing up for themselves every day. They have to choose to do that, and to care enough about themselves that they want that. From that place, they will be able to start showing up for themselves a little more each day. Soon enough, as they get better at meeting their own needs and ensuring they are pouring from a full cup, they will achieve the ability to love, connect, and serve so many more people than before, when they were pouring from an empty cup.

So, when you're communicating with another human, that's your opportunity to test your boundaries and practice your inner focus. To smooth and steady your energy and get it right within yourself. When you are in an interaction with another person, you can simultaneously interact with them *and* give yourself permission to tune in to how you feel about the interaction.

If you and I are having a conversation, I would want you to maintain your own practice, even as you are listening to me. That is, while I'm talking to you, I want you to ask yourself, "Am I inside my body as Kelsey is talking to me? How comfortable am I right now? Am I breathing? Where am I, in this moment of Kelsey talking to me? How am I feeling right now?" This will help you to shift into a state of association of self rather than a state of disassociation of self where you feel that other person's way, energy, needs, demands, ego. Even when the interaction is positive and warm and wonderful, you can still be checking in with yourself to monitor how *you* are feeling, as you talk together.

This can make some people feel guilty. They think they always have to help. Actually, this is a way to help others without interfering or controlling. You do not always have to help. Trust yourself. Maybe you see somebody who's really sad and you think you should go over and try to make them feel better, but you check in with yourself and you recognize that you really don't feel like approaching that person or you just don't have the energy in that moment. That's okay. You don't need to go over there. It might be that the sad person needs that time alone in their sadness in order to move through it. Who are you to say that it's your job to help them out of their sadness? You can't possibly have that information, so instead, trust your body and your intuition and act on what you feel compelled to do, not what you think you should do.

When you find this hard to do, you can tap into Reiki (I'll show you how to do this later in this chapter), so you have a channel of light in your body that can protect you from taking on energy that isn't yours to carry or help you to share light in a way that feels supportive to you, too. This will allow you to step out into the world with a sense of love and light, knowing that others might feel better just seeing your smile, without you needing to actively give by doing.

To help you begin awakening your own relation-ing, here are seven questions to think about. Answer them, either in your mind or in your journal, as they apply to any relationship you think needs new energy or needs to become more interdependent:

1. *When you are with this person, do you feel like yourself, or do you feel as if you are someone else within the relationship than you are outside the relationship?*

2. *Does this person make you feel any negative emotions about yourself, or does this person make you feel proud of who you are?*

3. *Does the energy between you and this person feel balanced or one-sided? If you aren't sure, ask yourself how you feel when you say goodbye and walk away from that person. Do you feel depleted or energized?*

4. *Do either you or this person tell the other what to do or try to control the other person's words, actions, or decisions? Do either of you criticize or undermine the other person's behaviors or actions to try to get them to change?*

5. *Do you trust and feel supported by this person, or do you feel that you or they withhold information or emotions due to mistrust or fear of a lack of support?*

6. *When you disagree, how does the energy feel to you? List some words to describe it.*

7. *When you are away from this person, do you feel better, worse, more whole, less whole, relieved, sad, or exactly the same, even though you enjoy being with them and look forward to being with them again?*

This practice of checking in with yourself will help you to fine-tune your intuition so you can make better relationship decisions. You'll begin to notice that when you interact with certain people, you feel present and good in your body, and when you interact with other people, you notice tension, physical pain, a sudden headache, or just a general sense of discomfort in your body. Those are messages from you to yourself, guiding you toward and away from certain relationships.

Maybe it's just that you need to take a break from interacting with someone for a while. That might be exactly the right thing for you to do. There have been countless students and clients I've worked with over the years who have family members, friends, or partners they are afraid of setting boundaries with, so they end up suffering very deep pain. They remain in the relationship because they are too scared to say (or to admit to themselves) that they no longer want to have a relationship with that person. I've experienced this firsthand myself. While setting boundaries may feel incredibly hard, I also know that none of us can make another person care about their own well-being or even their own life, and none of us can ever truly control the choices of another. Even if the other person is suffering as a result of their own actions, and you keep trying to help, they won't change until they decide to change. It's not up to you. You need to speak your truth and meet yourself right where you are in your needs. This is more than enough—it is where your responsibility ends.

There are also times when your body messages are so strong that you recognize your need to end a relationship. On the other side of this hard choice is freedom, joy, and a sense of self that you've likely not known for a long time. Through these experiences and your willingness to be honest with yourself, you may also recognize who you genuinely and authentically want to spend more time with, and which relationships you want to nurture consciously. But even in these positive states, stay in that place of awareness with yourself. Remind yourself: "I can help this person, but only if they participate because they want to help themselves, and I'm going to keep checking in with myself to make sure I'm meeting my needs first. I get to be my most important friend and client." That is the single most vital state to maintain if you want to be good at relation-ing.

When you meet yourself in all your needs and with all your own imbalances, balances, and everything in between, you can turn on that inner knowing for the sake of your own joy and harmony each day, and you can go out into the world in all your fullness. When you have met your own needs and you are aware of where you are and are not in balance, you will become luminous with that fullness. Others will see you and feel your energy and they may think, "I want what that person has." You're not doing the work for them, but you are beaming out energy that can make others want to find their own fullness. This is how you can create space for other people to meet their own needs and thrive better in their own relationships, whether with you or in their other interactions. You can become someone else's light, and they can choose to be inspired by it, or they can choose not to be. Either way, you've done what you need to do to burn bright for you and your well-being. What others choose to see or do with that is none of your business.

The need for connection and relationships isn't reserved for humans. If you have ever seen a dog who has been alone in a kennel for many hours, then gets let out to greet its people, or you've seen the way a zoo animal acts if it is alone in a cage, you can see how desperately animals crave connection. When animals are isolated, they develop many of the same problems humans do. They show signs of depression, anxiety, aggression, self-harm, even psychosis, from mice and rats who attack each other or binge on sugar or drugs[10] to polar bears that swim in figure eights for hours without stopping and parrots who pluck out all their own feathers.[11]

But even though animals seek out animals and people seek out people, we can help each other out. Imagine being alone in a room for hours. Now imagine being alone in a room for hours . . . with a friendly dog or an affectionate cat. Research shows that people who are lonely, depressed, or anxious feel much better when they have a pet to take care of. One study revealed that among single women who live alone, having a pet significantly reduced feelings of loneliness.[12] A bond with another being is a bond with another being—it can be physically, mentally, and spiritually rewarding. But if you don't have a pet or don't want a pet, you can still observe animals in the natural world and appreciate and have compassion for them. We're not so different from our animal friends.

CREATING CONNECTIONS

If you feel as if your relationships aren't so much the problem as the lack of them, then you may feel compelled to create more connections. It's easy to get into a habit of being alone or only interacting with a few people, but creating takes energy, which will build and brighten your own. Remember that we are social beings. Even if you need your alone time (and many of us do), your soul also craves connection with that web of energy—with other people, with other groups, with communities, and with something greater than yourself.

You may be connecting more than you think already. Consider all the ways that you already come together with people—or the opportunities you have that would allow you to make connections, forge a friendship, be part of a social group, or engage in a community. There are holidays, weddings, showers, and birthdays. There are book groups and dinner parties, community events like festivals and fairs, and the everyday casual connections friendly people make passing each other on the street with a smile, a nod, a "good morning" (especially in smaller towns).

You might participate in some of these things, but you can certainly choose to connect with other people more. You can decide to go to new events, go to places where people are, take a community class, or get involved in any other activities where you will meet people. It's easy to get into the habit of staying home and not doing something, but if you feel a lack of energy from not having social connections in your life, getting out there is your medicine.

Think about all the ways you could create connections. You could go to a retreat—maybe a yoga or meditation retreat, or a workshop or a retreat based on something you love to do, like biking, wine tasting, travel, bird-watching . . . whatever it is. You could meet people who also love to do the same thing. There are cooking clubs and gardening clubs, hiking groups and fitness classes and art classes and meet-ups of local people with all kinds of common interests. When I owned Pure Barre studios, many of our clients loved coming to classes together throughout the week and meeting up for coffee after class. Many of them said it was their favorite way to spend a weekend. You could start going to a running club or a meditation center. You could start a regular rotating discussion group of friends who want to talk about current events, or a monthly moon ritual circle at your home (see pages 263–266), or a jam session with people who all play different instruments. I have regular dinner parties in our home because it fills me with joy and a feeling of love and support that I don't get in other places. Rather than waiting for it to happen, I decided long ago that I would just create the connections myself. People in this digital age are hungry for real face-to-face connection, even if they don't know it, and a good meal and a glass of wine with friends can help.

But to find people, you have to be willing to participate in something new. In her TED Talk, Dr. Pinker theorizes that the reason women live longer than men is that they actively seek out social connections more than men do. I once heard a saying that the healthiest thing men can do is be married, and the healthiest thing women can do is have a close group of female friends. But I know men need social groups beyond their spouses. Otherwise, that is a lot of need put onto one person, and I believe men truly crave that connection with other men as well.

My husband is a very introverted guy, so I suggested that he start a dinner group with his guy friends. They now go out to a new restaurant once a month and it has become the most fun, therapeutic, joyful thing for all of them. They are all very different, but they each love this wonderful new connection in their lives. They laugh and joke and tease each other, and I predict that the positive energy they generate from this wonderful new ritual will keep them all alive and healthier for longer than they would be otherwise.

Creating connections isn't always easy, and one of the main reasons I've found that people hesitate to put themselves out there is a fear of vulnerability. And yet, one of the most beautiful things you can experience in a relationship is the ability to be vulnerable. When was the last time you truly shared from the depths of your heart, perhaps even the depths of your fears, with someone you love? When was the last time you really allowed yourself to be afraid, to be insecure, or to admit the intimate parts of your being to another person? Do you know how it feels to be that open with someone else? Many of my students say they never have been, but this is what you can do when you have genuine support from someone else who exists in their own fullness.

Relationships with others have energetic power, and when friendships and groups form and connections start, that's when the magic happens. A group of people can generate energy beyond any one person, and when they use that energy with intention, it's transformative.

You can see this in stories (and research) about the power of prayer. Alfred, Lord Tennyson wrote, "More things are wrought by prayer than this world dreams of." It's difficult to prove that prayer works, but a lot of people have tried to verify and demonstrate that prayer, meditation, and Reiki healing sent to people from a distance can actually have an effect. One thing we know for sure is that prayer helps the person who prays.

Ask someone who has experienced the power of prayer firsthand and you will likely get a passionate answer. When you are part of a community and you can ask for support, prayers, healing energy, or whatever you believe will help you, of course you will feel more supported, feel less stressed, and enjoy all the benefits I've already told you about that come with social connections. But when you receive this energy from others, I think it goes beyond just knowing you have support. When I'm going through a difficult time, I ask my closest friends to send me light and energy or love and healing, and I've experienced how completely my energy and my mind and my entire day shift.

One of my close friends is an incredible singer. She went on tour right after having a baby. We would talk regularly because as she was on tour, I was also in the midst of a full schedule and working on this book. There were many days when one of us was depleted and we would reach out to the other one and send each other prayers throughout the course of several months, when we were both going through very demanding times in our lives. And it worked! I would send her prayers and Reiki and reminders of how she could just surrender and allow her higher self to come through and receive God's support, and she would do the same for me. It was beautiful and, more than anything, feeling the support of another human on the most real and vulnerable level was a true gift.

You may already have some ideas about what prayer is, but consider expanding your definition. To me, prayer is a concentration and direction of spiritual energy, and this energy is healing, whether you call your conscious spreading of that energy "prayer" or something else. Reiki, which I'll talk about a bit later in this chapter, is the intentional direction of this energy for healing, and it can have intense healing power. To me, it is its own sort of prayer, and I've witnessed it working in a similar way. After hearing about how many people felt that they didn't have a community to rely upon, I decided to create an online Facebook Reiki group for people who were interested in Reiki and seeking community. It's called Reiki Healer's Society (you're welcome to join us!), and recently one of our members had a baby. The baby was having some health complications and had been in the NICU for two weeks, with no sign of improvement. The mom was frantic. She asked our Reiki group to send Reiki energy to her baby, and that night, we all, in our separate locations, sent out distance Reiki to that baby. The very next morning, doctors said the baby was doing much better and was okay to go home that day. The very next day!

Obviously a newborn baby couldn't know we were sending Reiki. You couldn't attribute that to the placebo effect or social support. I can't prove it, but I believe that intentional healing energy made the difference. There are countless stories just like this, but instead of just hearing them from others, I want you to try it in your own life!

~~~~~

THE ENERGY THAT CONNECTS US

So what is this energy, exactly? Let's take a moment to talk again about life-force energy, or universal energy, or ki, or chi, or prana. This energy goes by many names, but people have been aware of it and have been naming it for thousands of years.

This divine energy is like a higher intelligence that moves through us in every moment. When you connect to the breath in yoga, you are connecting to this energy. When you activate Reiki, you are connecting to this energy. It's like a pulsing-ness inside of you, and, intuitively, you know it's there. You've felt it. You might not feel it all the time, and that's okay, but you've felt it at some point, even if you didn't know that was what you were feeling.

According to ancient systems of health, like traditional Chinese medicine and Ayurveda, energy moves throughout the human body along tens of thousands of channels—in yoga we call them *nadis*—in certain directions, and it has little waystations throughout the body that are roughly associated with nerve centers. These centers are all over the body and they are called chakras. Different traditions place them and name them in slightly different ways, but these are the seven that people most often hear about and work with:

1. **ROOT CHAKRA:** *The first chakra,* Muladhara, *is at the base of your spine. Its color association is red. This chakra contains the energy that heals your structural body, and gives you a sense of security, safety, and groundedness.*

2. **SACRAL CHAKRA:** *The second chakra,* Swadisthana, *is located around the navel. Its color association is orange. This chakra contains the energy of creativity, sexuality, and emotions.*

3. **SOLAR PLEXUS CHAKRA:** *The third chakra,* Manipura, *is in the area beneath the breastbone, between the two lower sides of the rib cage. Its color association is yellow. This is where the energy of life purpose, emotions, and strength of will originate.*

4. **HEART CHAKRA:** *The fourth chakra,* Anahata, *is behind the heart. Its color association is green. This is the center of romantic love, altruism, generosity, and loving-kindness.*

5. **THROAT CHAKRA:** *The fifth chakra,* Vishuddha, *is located in the hollow of the throat. Its color association is blue. It contains the energy of communication, speech, speaking your truth, and intelligence.*

6. **THIRD-EYE CHAKRA:** *The sixth chakra,* Ajna, *is located just above the point between the eyebrows. Its color association is indigo. It is the center of spiritual perception, wisdom, and intuition.*

7. **CROWN CHAKRA:** *The seventh chakra,* Sahasrara, *is located at or just above the crown of the head. Its color association is violet. It is the chakra that takes in spiritual energy from a higher source. This is where we communicate with spirit and this is where we access energy for Reiki healing.*

There are many ways to work with the chakras, and I'll give you a chakra meditation to try on pages 272–276, but when you open yourself to awareness, you may be able to feel the energy in these chakras, and beyond them, throughout your body, as energy moves and flows. You can also feel where it's leaking out or blocked. An energy leak results in an area that is too low in energy, and usually feels depleted, and an energy block results in an area that feels stagnant. Either one is a disharmony and leads to imbalance, which may have negative effects in the body, mind, or spirit.

The blockage could feel like physical pain, or a foggy spot, or a dark spot that feels stagnant and still inside of you. A leak could feel like an emptiness, draining, or a sense of fatigue. It could be that you feel dissociated with a certain part of your body, or it could manifest as an emotion or an excess of feeling, such as anger, anxiety, or sadness. Wherever you feel a disharmony, that is an energy leak or an energy block.

Energy blocks can also exist in your home, if you feel a disharmony in a certain area of your living space. It could be in your job, or in a relationship. Think about what parts of your life don't feel right, or feel in disharmony, and you will get a sense of where those blockages and leaks are happening. I feel energy leaks when I get too busy and forget to do those basic things for myself that I know I need. If I rush off in the morning without doing my morning ritual, or I grab my phone right away and start answering emails before I even get a chance to have a glass of water, I'm creating energy leaks. When I feel them, that's when I know I'm going to have to get in there like a spiritual plumber and repair them.

CHECK-IN TIME:

Let's take a moment so that you can pause and check in with yourself. Take some deep breaths and focus inward. How are you feeling? Don't judge, just notice.

TEACHERS, COACHES, MENTORS, GUIDES, AND GURUS

If you get interested in energy practices and energy healing, you will probably seek out a teacher or a guide at some point. I don't know where I would be without the teachers, mentors, and guides who have helped me along the way. You can learn a lot about your own spiritual practice through a teacher, but it's also important for you not to give your power away. A teacher is there to guide you into your own power, not to take over your life. Not every teacher will know what is best for you, and no teacher knows you better than you know yourself. If you ever feel a deep resistance to something a teacher tells you to do, listen to your intuition. You don't ever have to be at the mercy of another human being. Even if you deeply admire a teacher, be aware of how that relationship works, so it doesn't slip into idolatry. No teacher is perfect. We are all human beings, just like you—even the most famous ones.

There are some ways to tell if a teacher, health coach, mentor, or guide is qualified to instruct or advise you. The most important thing in my opinion is that the teacher has their own at-home practice. A yoga or meditation teacher who is not also refining and continually learning and practicing doesn't have the deep internal connection to keep guiding others. A health coach who doesn't follow their own advice is not necessarily qualified to advise others. Every teacher, coach, mentor, guide, and guru should also be willing to look at their own imperfections and own their own human-ness. And I will add that if you choose to be a teacher, coach, or guide in this world, I hope that you will continue to have your own inner practice, do your own inner work, and keep a perspective about who you are and what kind of teachings you are sharing with others.

Finally, at some point, every teacher-student relationship comes to an end. There is a saying that when the student is ready, the teacher appears. I also like to say that when the student is ready, the teacher disappears. We all have teachers and mentors who are right for different times in our lives, and they are beautiful gifts, but when an attachment to a teacher keeps you from moving forward or growing, or when you start depending on that teacher too much, it may be time to move on.

I was very dependent on my Reiki master. I remember once when I left the dinner table while on vacation with my husband just to take a phone call from her. When we parted ways, I felt lost and confused and almost incapable of knowing what to do or where to go in my life. In hindsight, I see that ending that relationship was necessary. It didn't exactly end well, although it didn't exactly end dramatically, either. But, ultimately, her presence was a gift, and the end of our connection was also a beautiful gift because I had to learn how to go out on my own, and I never could have done that if I had stayed attached to her guidance.

REIKI AND THE CHANNELING OF ENERGY TO LIGHT UP YOUR LIFE

I've saved the best for last—Reiki, my favorite and most cherished practice. Reiki is the therapy that I once thought was ridiculous, that I didn't believe in, that I knew couldn't be real. And it's the healing practice that has made the most difference in my life, more than anything else I've done. I'm so excited for you to feel the power and presence of the energy within you and to learn how to concentrate that energy for greater healing for yourself. To practice Reiki is to allow yourself the honor of becoming a channel for energy in the service of healing yourself and, eventually—if you undergo the training and have a desire and feel full from doing your own healing work on yourself—to heal others.

The question I get asked more than any other is this: "What is Reiki?" A lot of people are curious about this seemingly mysterious but actually very practical energy-healing technique. Reiki can become a personal practice as you learn to work with your own energy. My Reiki master once said that Reiki is "exercises designed as deliberate footsteps toward absorbing your small ego and realigning with your highest self."

Reiki is a Japanese word. *Rei* means "God's wisdom or higher power" and *ki* means "life-force energy," so *Reiki* literally means spiritually guided life-force energy or universal life-force energy. It is pronounced RAY-key. As I shared before, each of us has thousands of energy channels all over the body, and we have more than one hundred chakras inside us, including a chakra in the palm of each hand. This is the place where we connect the energy to bring about healing, through whatever you (or the person you are healing) needs, and the intention of Reiki is always balance and harmony.

If you've ever taken a yoga class, you may have heard of prana. If you've ever had acupuncture or learned tai chi, you have probably heard of chi. Prana and chi are the same thing as ki. They all refer to universal life-force energy. Reiki, like yoga and acupuncture and tai chi, works by deliberately aligning and connecting with this energy, balancing and harmonizing it in the body, mind, and spirit.

This energy is real, although it is not the focus of Western medicine. My teacher once told me that Reiki is the "bio-photon (light) emission conducted from one organic species to another." It is a fact that humans emit energy, and Reiki just takes this a step further, teaching practitioners to tune in to and move that energy and light in healing ways.

Reiki certainly has a mystical component. I've had several experiences both as a recipient of Reiki and as a practitioner that simply cannot be explained by logic. I'll often teach workshops around the country where I'll guide a meditation and then go around the room and conduct Reiki on each person. Sometimes there are more than seventy people in the room. Afterward, several of the students will come up to me and want to share or connect about their experiences. One woman may tell me that she was grateful for the Reiki because she immediately felt a cooling sensation on her very inflamed injured knee. What this means is that she needed balance and harmony in her knee to receive relief, and that is what she got from Reiki. The person who sat right next to her might say that they felt a perfect temperature of warmth that helped ease and relax their stiff neck. Another student may tell me they fell asleep and felt a deep sense of peace. Again, the effect was balancing. It's not because my hands or the temperature of my body had been changed—it's because, as I served as an open channel for life-force energy to come through me, these people were each able to receive whatever healing and alignment they needed.

Because I teach Reiki, I hear stories almost every day about how Reiki has transformed people's lives, in great ways and in small ways. People have upended their entire lives and used Reiki to surrender to the joys of the unknown, like my student Bella, who quit her high-powered job in fashion marketing to become a yoga teacher. At first she wondered if she had made a terrible mistake, but then she took a Reiki Level 1 class, just to add to her knowledge of energy healing and enhance her yoga practice. What she found was a method by which she could find true courage within herself to change a life that drained her into a life that filled her up. She says she never would have made it without Reiki. She would have gotten scared and given up, but Reiki filled her with the light and the support she needed to see the path forward.

A good friend of mine was never trained in Reiki, but I showed her how to do Reiki on herself and now she tells me that she always uses it before important business meetings or phone calls where she needs to be clearheaded, calm, and unafraid. She says that when she uses Reiki to fill herself up with light, or to fill up the room before a big meeting, the meetings or calls always go well—and often much better than she would have dreamed.

Many of my students use Reiki every day to manage anxiety or to prompt healing in their own bodies. They use it to infuse themselves for the day, so they can walk into the world feeling supported, balanced, excited, expansive, and open to the possibilities of the unknown. Reiki has helped many people, myself included, move through pain, and also move through the knee-jerk reactions of their own egos. A dear friend of mine used Reiki to help her put up a boundary between herself and someone who was holding her back in life in some very negative ways. She felt she would never be able to untangle herself from this person, but Reiki suddenly made it feel possible. She was able to find and honor herself again.

Learning to channel Reiki energy for your own healing isn't complicated. (I'll walk you through it on pages 230–233.) Anyone can do it. The power is within all of us. Reiki can become a part of your life as you learn to work with your own energy and the energy all around you. It may be one of the most potent tools you have for achieving greater self-awareness and understanding the nature of your true self, beneath all your imprints and emotions and health issues. Reiki can wake you up and raise your awareness about what is no longer serving your highest good, so you can live more authentically and with a sense of divine connection and guidance.

Once you become comfortable with Reiki energy, you can infuse it into anything around you. At home, I reiki my food so I can best receive its nourishment and support. I'll reiki my computer if I'm going to be sending out an important email (or writing this book!). I reiki my plants so they will thrive, and I reiki my car before I get in it to drive somewhere. There are endless ways to work with this energy, and each person will find the ways to use it in their own life.

At first, it's normal to resist this practice. You might feel skeptical about it, as I did when I first heard about it. Or you may think you just don't have that kind of power or access inside of you. It is true that healing comes very naturally to certain people. There are those who tell me that sometimes their hands feel warm and they feel that they have some kind of healing ability. One student said that when she puts her hands over her dog, she feels like her hands heat up, even though she is not Reiki-trained. Another student told me that she has always been told that she has "healing hands." I don't doubt these stories because I know there is an innate ease of access for some people—they have a natural gift for letting Reiki energy flow through them.

But I want you to know that even if you think you can't "do Reiki," there is no barrier. I would never have thought I would be a Reiki healer, especially when I was working in the US Senate. No way! But as I learned over time, and as you are hopefully learning or being reminded of now, Reiki (or prana or chi) is everywhere, all around you and within you, and all around and within everyone and everything all the time. We can use our life-force energy for good if we choose. To use it only involves becoming aware of it and being willing to use it. Don't be discouraged if you try the Reiki practices in this book and they don't feel the way you think they will, or the way others have described the experience. Everyone experiences the energy flow differently, so please don't judge yourself or think you are doing it wrong. There is no wrong way to Reiki or meditate or connect with yourself! You are showing up for you each time you do any of these practices, and that's what matters, and that is exactly what will begin to bring about the big shifts. We all have a very unique and individual life experience and journey, and your experience is yours, and it is perfect.

Once you learn Reiki, you may also forget that you have it as a tool in your life. My students often message me to say, "I'm supersick!" or "I'm so stressed about this upcoming presentation!" or "I have this big event!" and I will answer, "Did you Reiki yourself?" They are often surprised. They forgot they could do that! I tell them to Reiki themselves before messaging me to send them Reiki, and see what shifts on their own. It won't hurt to give it a try, and it could change your life. Many of my students have gone on to experience major life transformations because of Reiki, and many have become practitioners themselves. No matter what is happening, Reiki first!

✦ THE SCIENCE OF REIKI ✦

There is actually some science behind Reiki. According to Bernadette Doran, who contributed to the student manual I use in my Reiki Level 1 training at the DEN Meditation Center in Los Angeles, one of the most basic laws of physics, Ampere's Law, explains the nature of electrical and magnetic energies in and around the human body and how electrical currents flow through conductors like the human body. This creates a magnetic field around the body and has been measured (by Dr. John Zimmerman) coming out of the hands of Reiki therapists, in the same frequency ranges that are optimal for stimulating healing.

For those of you who are still skeptical, I also encourage trust. The beauty of Reiki is that you don't need to understand how it works. You only need to trust that it works. Drop out of your logic and into your spirit. Reiki is something to feel, not something to analyze. The more you practice it, the more your life will change and the more you will heal and progress toward self-actualization. When you connect to the Reiki source, you are like a firefighter holding the fire hose. It's the water that is doing the work—the life-force energy—and you are simply the one holding the hose and directing the energy of the water.

To help guide you as you seek to bring Reiki into your life, here are the Reiki precepts, which are a summary of the teachings of Mikao Usui, the founder of Reiki. They have become touchstones for Reiki practitioners as they harmonize themselves for healing. You can use them in any way you like—as affirmations, as part of meditation, or as guidelines for how to live your life. Practicing these five precepts can help put your energy in the right place for practicing Reiki. You can find many different translations and versions of these precepts, but this is the way I teach them:

1. *Just for today, do not worry.*

2. *Just for today, do not anger.*

3. *Just for today, be humble.*

4. *Just for today, be honest.*

5. *Just for today, be compassionate toward yourself and others.*

Although we don't really know all the history of where Reiki came from, we do know that it has been modernized (as yoga has) for twenty-first-century use. The Reiki we do and the Reiki I teach are not exactly the same as the original Reiki, even though we retain much of the early philosophy, such as the Reiki precepts. Like every spiritual practice, Reiki has evolved. Centuries ago, none of the yoga masters could have envisioned yoga in a studio with hot air blowing in on purpose, with a Drake playlist and yoga mats and tight yoga pants! It's the same with Reiki. We are learning about Reiki here in modern times in a very Westernized and digestible way. The original methods were much more intense and complex, but what we do now is how Reiki works in this time and this place, and that is perfect because Reiki exists in the now and we exist in the now. How beautiful and lucky we all are to have access to this wonderful gift of self-healing.

YOUR REIKI PRACTICE

If you choose to start practicing Reiki, or especially if you choose to study Reiki with a Reiki master, you will do some intense internal work. Realigning your life will bring up a lot of stuff to work through—in the best, most loving way, but it will still be a process and your inner resources must go to self-healing, self-awareness, and increasing your own inner brightness before you can use those resources to heal others. Hone your ability to meet yourself in your own needs and in your own desires. Dig into your imprints, your fears, your loneliness, your pain, your anxiety, your disconnects. Go through it all, so you can come out on the other side, where you are healed and full of the light you need to become who you really are.

You can start that practice by waking up every morning and saying, "How am I going to allow myself to receive love today?" As you slide love back into your soul, you will open up the weaker, atrophied parts of yourself that have been dormant beneath your tail chasing, always-doing, and energetic stuckness. Love will light up all those dark corners you have inside that you have forgotten are in there. Your joy, your potential, your purpose, and your abilities will be bottomless.

CHECK-IN TIME:

Let's take a moment so that you can pause and check in with yourself. Take some deep breaths and focus inward. How are you feeling? Don't judge, just notice.

ARE YOU A HEALER?

Many people who experience Reiki immediately want to learn how to use it so they can become practitioners. If you feel this, it is very important to understand the importance of healing yourself before you start healing others. You have to learn what it feels like to feel this energy. You have to learn what it feels like to intuit where your hands go next. You have to learn how to feel a deepness in the energy, and also how to feel when you are not as connected. You have to learn to pull your hands back when the energy is too strong, and get closer when you need to concentrate the energy more. You need to give yourself the space to practice with yourself and, most important, to honor yourself and the journey of going inward and giving yourself space to do the healing needed before supporting others.

People tend to attract others into their lives who have the same issues as they do. Other people are our mirrors, and they can be amazing healing allies because they help us see what it is we need to bring to the light. For that reason, in this journey, you must focus on your own healing and awareness first. Get clear and aligned with love, and then you can help others from that aware and loving space.

That being said, we are all human, so don't attempt to be "perfect" or "completely healed" before starting to train in Reiki, if you feel called to do that. If you do, begin with Reiki Level 1. Next, in Reiki Level 2, you will do a lot of deep work of healing your past with distance Reiki (sending Reiki across space or time), and learn how to start healing others. Reiki Level 2 can dig up a lot of emotional healing for people, and it takes surrender to get through it. Next is Reiki Level 3, and then Reiki Master Teacher. If you complete Reiki Master Teacher, you will be at the level to pass on the lineage and teach others how to practice Reiki.

But Reiki isn't a contest. It's not about certifying yourself to these new levels so that you can be bigger and better. If you only take a Reiki 1 class, you can learn enough to help you for the rest of your life. You don't have to go on to the other levels to get very good at working on yourself. If you choose to just use the Reiki shared in this book for yourself, that is enough. It's for you to intuit.

Innately, we all have some desire to go out and help others, to be capable and distinctive in the world, and to be sharing and loving. We all want to find the biggest, brightest expression of ourselves in the external world, but if you don't go inward to find all that light, all that delight—if you're looking out there to find something that is within, you're going to come up empty-handed. There's nothing that I can do for you that's going to give that to you. Only you can turn the light on inside yourself. All I can do is point you toward your own magic. And then one day, you're going to wake up, and you're going to be there. Believe in yourself. You're going to love how that feels.

~~~~~

SURRENDER TO THE FLOW

At its essence, moving with the flow of energy in a way that is natural and harmonized requires a certain level of surrender. Just as surrender is necessary in life, surrender is necessary in Reiki. Have you ever watched someone whitewater rafting? Some people struggle and look terrified and fight it, and others seem to navigate the rough rapids with perfect calm. They move around the rocks and over the falls with ease, as if they were nothing. These are the people who are moving with the flow of energy, and this can be a metaphor for how you move with energy in your own life. Instead of fighting the currents, like those people who can barely stay in their raft, you can choose to practice the art and beauty of surrender. Let the energy guide you.

Even if your life up to now has been one long struggle, one long fight, here you are right now, ready to feel the flow of energy in your own life. You got here, and that is what matters. When you choose a willingness to be aware, to acknowledge what is true, to accept and feel the energy of life and how it flows, then you won't have to effort so hard anymore.

Every day, ask yourself: *Where can I give myself permission to surrender? Where can I give myself permission to receive and be fully connected to myself and to my life?* You can recognize when somebody wants you to do something you don't want to do, and you can choose to surrender to that energy of not-doing. Where are you fighting? Where are you striving? Where are you effort-ing, trying to do all these things you've decided are so necessary? Are they really so necessary that you would suffer because of them? Where do you want to thrive *now*? Where, in your day-to-day life, can you stop and think, *Okay. Someone wants me to do this, but I want to do something else. I'm going to put my request of myself into the equation and make my decision with my own needs factored in.* Right?

Maybe that looks like agreeing to meet a friend, but only for fifteen minutes to touch base. You don't have to explain yourself. You don't have to say what else you need to be doing, or make up some white lie so your excuse sounds more urgent to someone else. You can just start to practice your truth and show up for yourself, and see how amazing that feels. The more you release, the more you feel safe in releasing. Even if you can say, "For five seconds, I'm going to feel what it feels like not to have this imprint that I am not the smart one," or "For five seconds, I'm going to feel what it feels like if I didn't have this job," or "For five seconds, I'm going to feel what it feels like to be totally in love with everything around me," that is a beginning. The more you practice that, the more ease you will feel. Just like anything else—just like meditation or breathwork or doing Reiki on yourself— you get better with practice. Practice surrender, forgive yourself for your mistakes, and give yourself permission to experience your own life and live in your own space, maybe with a little gratitude for what you have right now.

But always remember the importance of connection. Meeting your own needs also means reaching out to the people who are there for you and asking for help when you need it. It's okay to say, "Hey, can you send me some extra prayers today or some love, or can you send some healing my way?" Even if you've never done Reiki, you can always direct your love and energy with intention toward other people, other things, other situations.

Awareness of yourself is the key and serenity is the gift of surrendering.

At its heart, spiritual health is you, surrendering. It's you, learning that life is something bigger than you that you don't need to control. It's you, living in the awareness of the present moment. You can let energy, and feelings, and love, and light, and life itself flow and move through you without needing to know how or why it works. You can let Reiki move through you and remind you to surrender, that you have the ability of letting go, of not controlling, of being in that raft and moving over the rapids as if you've been doing it your whole life. Practice Reiki. Practice surrender. Practice awareness. Practice acceptance of you in this moment, right now. The more you do it, the more you stop doubting and questioning and controlling, and the more you allow yourself to have access to this clear channel that is your birthright, the more amazing your life will become.

Let this idea of surrender and trust sink in, and then you will be ready to try some Reiki.

~~~~~

LEARNING TO FEEL THE REIKI ENERGY

Before you can start using Reiki, you need to learn how to feel the Reiki energy that is within you. At the beginning, it's a good idea to do this practice daily. The more you practice channeling this energy, the quicker and easier it will be to turn it on. Even though Reiki energy is constantly going in and out of you, just as the universe is constantly ready to support and help you, what you are learning to do is to consciously turn it on and awaken to it and feel it. So make this exercise a routine part of your day and you will build your awareness like a muscle. Before you know it, the connection will be so strong, it will always be there when you need it. Because this ritual is best performed with your eyes closed, I recommend listening to the audio version of this book, or recording yourself reading it.

Here's how to begin:

1. *Find a comfortable seated position. Place your hands into a prayer position, honor yourself and your willingness to be open and to heal, and honor the Reiki energy you will channel through this process. You can also say this out loud: "I honor myself. I honor the sacred healing of Reiki. Let me be a channel for divine energy, for my highest good and the highest good of all beings."*

2. *Put your hands on your legs, palms facing up. Begin by taking a few deep breaths. Leave your eyes open if you desire. When you begin to feel settled, close your eyes and allow the breath to move through your body.*

3. *Visualize a beautiful bright light energy above you. Inhale and envision that light moving into the crown of your head and down into your heart. Inhale and exhale slowly and deeply a few times, envisioning the bright light continuing to pour in through your crown and go down through your head, your throat, and then allow it to fill up your heart with clear, divine, healing energy.*

4. *Continue to inhale the light into your heart, but now, with each exhalation, envision that light moving from your heart out into your entire body, down your arms and into your hands, down your legs and into your feet, filling up every single cell and sweeping the energy along with it.*

5. *Continue to breathe in this way, inhaling the light through your crown and into your heart, exhaling the light out into your entire body. Feel the light becoming warm and healing. Do this for a few minutes.*

6. *Next, as you continue to inhale light, begin to concentrate the movement of your exhalation so the light moves from your heart down your arms and into your palms. Let the energy concentrate there. Breathe in the light, breathe it out into your palms. Feel the energy accumulating in the palms of your hands.*

7. *When you feel that you can really feel that energy in your palms, place your hands over your heart and imagine the stream of light moving from your palms right back into your body, through the heart, in a loop or a circuit. You may imagine this visually or feel the warmth or even hear the sound of the flowing energy from your crown to your heart to your palms and back into your heart. There is no wrong way to feel this energy. Stay this way, continuing to experience the warm light moving in this pattern, or whatever pattern comes through for you. If you need a vision, imagine light coming into the crown, into the heart, out the palms, and back into the heart. This is the essence of Reiki.*

8. *When you feel that you are ready, slowly bring your hands close together. Do you feel the energy between them? Stay here as long as you need to. It's okay if you don't feel anything specific. There is no right or wrong here. Then, bring your palms together into a prayer position. Take a moment to thank the Reiki, and yourself, and the teacher within you, and the healer within you.*

9. *When you feel ready, gently move your arms and legs, then your fingers and toes. Feel yourself coming back into the space where you are sitting.*

10. *Open your eyes when you are ready. Get up and drink some water, maybe have something light to eat so you can get back into your body. Or, you could use a grounding or awakening essential oil, but stay in silence for the next few minutes. You may want to journal about this experience after you are done. Do so in silence, honoring this space you have created for yourself and your own healing.*

✦ IT'S NOT YOU, IT'S REIKI ✦

It's important to remember that you are not the one doing Reiki. You are opening yourself up to be a vessel and a channel to that life-force energy, from universal consciousness and healing energy coming in through your crown chakra and out through your palm chakras. You are only the delivery system.

HOW TO USE YOUR REIKI

Now that you have a practice for feeling Reiki energy, you can begin to use that energy for specific purposes. Really, you can use Reiki for anything. You can use it for physical healing, emotional healing, spiritual healing, to help alleviate feelings of anxiety or depression or burnout or overwhelm, to rejuvenate you when you are tired or relax you when you can't get to sleep, and so much more.

A student of mine recently wrote to me that she moved from California to Mexico and it was a very stressful move, but according to her email to me, Reiki saved her and her family, keeping them calm and grounded. When her child broke his finger, he asked her to reiki his finger on the way to the doctor's office, and it helped! In her new city, she was recently invited to lead a guided meditation at someone's home and ended up giving Reiki to one of Mexico's most powerful businessmen. And she has only taken my Reiki Level 1 class—I can only imagine what she will accomplish after she takes Reiki Level 2!

Personally, I use Reiki daily. I reiki my food, I reiki my home, my mail, or the checks I am sending out. You can use Reiki however you wish once you feel comfortable feeling the energy, but here are some exercises you might also want to try. For each of these exercises, start by doing the previous exercise to help you feel and channel Reiki energy. Or, if you already feel in tune with the energy, you can just say to yourself, "Turn Reiki on," or something similar, and go ahead with the following exercises.

~~~~~

REIKI FOR PAIN OR INJURY

If you are feeling physical pain somewhere in your body, or you have an injury that needs to heal, Reiki can help. If the pain or injury is acute, you only need to do this for a short time, such as two or three minutes, but it is useful to do it several times a day. Here's what to do:

1. *Sit or lie down and take a few deep breaths. When the Reiki energy is flowing, bring your hands to your heart and place your palms over your heart. Open yourself to support and guidance.*

2. *When your hands start to light up or feel heavy or warm, you are ready. If you aren't sure where the pain is coming from, move your palms to your forehead and ask (silently or out loud) to be shown where your body needs Reiki. You may see a body part or feel it or be shown the name of it, or you may just get a sense of what it is.*

KELSEY J. PATEL

3. *When you know (or if you already know) what part needs Reiki, just place your hands over that spot, either directly on it or hovering just above it, and go back to your breath pattern.*

4. *Keep breathing in light and allow it to move into your heart and down your arms and into the part of you that hurts or needs healing.*

5. *Ask for support and assistance to heal with ease and grace. Envision the light going into the place that needs healing, with flow and harmony.*

6. *After a few minutes, bring your hands back to your heart, take a few slow breaths, then open your eyes. Move slowly and respect your pain or injury by taking it easy and letting the Reiki energy work.*

~~~~~

REIKI FOR ANXIETY

Reiki is a powerful therapeutic tool for anxiety. Whenever I feel anxious, I like to do some tapping first (see page 167), to shake the anxious energy loose. Sometimes I cry and it begins releasing the anxiety and removing that sense of intense overwhelm. Then I do Reiki to release it. I recommend that you try three to five minutes of tapping first, and then do Reiki for about five minutes. For anxiety, you can do Reiki either sitting or lying down, depending on what feels most comfortable to you in the moment. Because this ritual is best performed with your eyes closed, I recommend listening to the audio version of this book, or recording yourself reading it. Here's what to do:

1. *Sit or lie down and take a few deep breaths. When the Reiki energy is flowing, bring your hands in front of your eyes and*

hover them there, gently moving them over the top and sides of your head. Feel the flow of light clearing the mind and its racing thoughts.

2. *Focus on your breath. Feel the calm, loving, energy light moving in through your crown, into your heart, down your arms, into your palms, and back into your head.*

3. *Do this for a minute or two, then bring your palms to your heart. Cup your hands over your heart, then gently press your palms into your chest while you say the words "Peace, peace, peace." Feel the words going into your heart.*

4. *When you begin to feel the anxiety subside, bring your hands to your knees and take a few more slow breaths before moving on with your day. Try to carry that sense of peace and inner quiet with you.*

～～～～

REIKI FOR EXHAUSTION

When you feel exhausted, fatigued, or just burned out, try Reiki, which will do whatever it is you need. If you need energy to make it through the rest of the day, Reiki will give you energy. If you need to calm yourself so you can finally get to sleep, Reiki will help you sleep. You might even fall asleep while you are doing it, which is totally fine. If you stay awake long enough, you can do Reiki for exhaustion longer than for other issues. I like to spend twenty minutes doing it. Because this ritual is best performed with your eyes closed, I recommend listening to the audio version of this book, or recording yourself reading it.

1. *Put on some comforting, relaxing music and lie down in a comfortable position.*

2. *Place your hands on your heart and allow your entire body to relax as much as you can.*

3. *Take some deep breaths and envision the light channeling either into the crown of your head or into the backs of your palms. If it helps, you can also imagine your angels or your guides directing the light into you. Or just say, "Turn Reiki on."*

4. *Let the light move into your heart and throughout your entire body, relaxing every muscle fiber and every cell. Really let your body release into healing.*

5. *When you feel relaxed and sleepy . . . go to sleep! Or, if you need to keep going, open your eyes and stretch and sit up, feeling renewed.*

〰️

REIKI YOUR FOOD

When I reiki my food, it's almost like saying grace. I usually add a prayer, but you can say or not say anything that feels right to you. When I am eating with friends, usually we all hold hands. I do this so often that now, when I sit down with friends, they all look at me expectantly and their kids sometimes say, "Let's do Aunt Kelsey's prayer!" I think it's a beautiful way to combine grace and Reiki to express appreciation and gratitude for the nourishment in front of you and all the ways it came to your table. Here's how I do it.

1. *Sit down at your table. Place your palms together and rub them a few times until you feel a bit of friction and warmth.*

2. *When you feel that energy, place your hands a few inches above your food and feel or say a blessing. I say this prayer: "Dear God, thank you for the food, the hands that have prepared it,*

and all the places that it has come from, to be at my table. I ask
that this food please nourish, sustain, and support my body."
You could also say something less specific, like, "I express my
gratitude for this food and the hands that have prepared it
and all the places it has come from, to be at my table. May it
nourish, sustain, and support my body."

3. *If I have friends or family present, we all hold hands and I*
might also add, "Thank you for this friendship, for the hearts
around the table, and for our health, happiness, love, and
continued abundance together."

~~~~~

REIKI YOUR PETS

Animals love Reiki and they are easy to reiki because they are so open to it. Animals I don't know often come up to me, as if they were asking for Reiki energy. Although I don't recommend that you reiki other people without some training, you can try doing Reiki on your pets. In your mind, always ask your animal's permission first, and if you get a sense that your animal is willing—they may even come to you from across the room—use the same method in the section on healing yourself to turn the Reiki on.

When you are ready to put your hands on or over the area to be healed, put them on or over your pet. Animals will often settle down, close their eyes, and soak it all in. Some will fall asleep. Animals are very sensitive, so they often prefer that you keep your hands above them but not on them. Others like you to touch them. The more you do this, the more you will get a feel for what your own pets prefer. Tune in to them and sense their energy, but let them take the lead.

Sessions with animals are usually shorter—usually just a few minutes. They will tell you when they are done by getting up and walking away or getting fidgety. Doing Reiki on animals regularly is good for them and it can also help you to feel more loving compassion and connection toward animals.

REIKI A LOVED ONE

If you are not technically trained in Reiki by working with a Reiki master to earn your certification, you are not intended to heal others as a profession, but you now know enough to offer Reiki healing and support to the people you love. What a beautiful way to spread goodness to your family and friends!

My family recently took a trip to Dubai. It was our first time there. On the second or third day, we were at a local farmers' market, and one of our sons wasn't feeling well. He looked pale and splotchy, and then suddenly he said that he couldn't breathe. Over the course of our vacation, we had to call an ambulance three separate times to take him to the hospital, where he spent several nights. For the sake of privacy, I won't go into detail except to say that the anxiety and panic this caused my son made his condition even worse. The only thing that helped him fall asleep each night was Reiki. Parents can feel helpless and scared about their child's health, safety, and well-being, and Reiki is a beautiful way to love and support your child's health and healing. It can benefit the entire family.

You can do Reiki on someone the same way you do it on yourself. The only two requirements are that you must ask for their permission to do Reiki, and never perform Reiki on someone if you or they are intoxicated in any way.

If you are going to do Reiki on a loved one, have them relax while you also relax and get the energy flowing. "Turn on" the Reiki. You may wish to hover your hands over their head at first and ask what they need. If you really tune in, you may feel where the energy is stuck or where the pain is. Move your hands to that area and place them over or on the area, depending on the comfort level of the person. Feel the energy flowing into the crown of your head, into your heart, down your arms, out your palms, and into the other person, filling them with warm healing light energy. If they ask you to stop, of course do so immediately. Otherwise, let them relax into a peaceful feeling and let the light and the Reiki energy move into them and work its magic. After you have spent five or ten minutes, gently remove your hands. You may want to hold their feet for a few minutes. When they are ready, they can slowly open their eyes.

You can also use Reiki to help others by sending it to them from a distance. Just imagine the Reiki healing moving into them. Or, you can reiki a space. If someone you love is in the hospital, or just at home feeling sick or sad, there may be a general sense of helplessness in the room, or coming from the people who want to help but don't know how. When you tap into the Reiki source, even if you have no idea what the outcome will be for that person, you can infuse their hospital room or home or bed or body with Reiki to bring balance and harmony. This can help to alleviate fear, pain, or whatever distress the person is feeling, and can bring a greater sense of peace into the environment.

Many of these techniques involve different levels of Reiki training and require different protocols. However, energy healing is available and intended for everyone. Once you start doing Reiki, I think you will find that there are opportunities to practice it everywhere. Use this powerful tool whenever you can. You may just find, as many of my students, clients, friends, and family members have found, that it changes your life.

CHECK-IN TIME:

Let's take a moment so that you can pause and check in with yourself. Take some deep breaths and focus inward. How are you feeling? Don't judge, just notice.

3

ROCK, PAPER, REIKI: RITUALS FOR A BRIGHT LIFE

CHAPTER EIGHT

Rock: Rituals for the Body

Ritual is the act of sanctifying action—even ordinary actions—so that it has meaning. I can light a candle because I need the light or because the candle represents the light I need.

—CHRISTINA BALDWIN, AMERICAN ACTOR AND WRITER

HUMANS HAVE BEEN practicing rituals for tens of thousands and maybe even millions of years. We have used rituals to worship the sun, the moon, the stars, the sky, and the divine forces we felt existed but could not see. We have used rituals to mark the changing of the days, the changing of the seasons, and the passing of the years. We have used rituals to mark births, the transition into adulthood, marriages, and deaths. We use rituals to find meaning in our lives and to mark the passing of our lives.

Rituals are very important to me. They are my reminder to come back to myself and to what really matters to me. They bring clarity. They help connect me to my heart, and they can do the same for you. Rituals can help you to notice where you've strayed too far from yourself, and what you need to do to come back to your center. They make life feel sacred again. Rituals have medicine for us, especially on a mental and psychological level. They connect us to our environments and to each other. In the world today, we don't revere rituals because we haven't been taught to revere them, but they can help us honor our own inner rhythms as they honor the rhythms and cycles of the natural world. In a time when people honor productivity and achievement, where people are always selling something, always going and doing, rituals provide a rest from that frenetic pace. It isn't natural to work without stopping. If you never stop and find a quiet space to honor the life you are living and feel your place in it, you will miss the most beautiful part of existence. Rituals are a sacred way to pause in awareness.

✦ ROCK, PAPER, REIKI ✦

One day, as I was meditating and connecting to my body, mind, and spirit, the idea of rock, paper, Reiki came to me. Remember that old children's game, Rock-Paper-Scissors? I used to play it all the time with my sister when we waited for brunch on Sunday after going to church with our parents and grandparents. For me, rock is the body—the physical substance, the groundedness, and the earth element of the world we live. Paper is the mind, the realm of thinking, writing, communicating, visualizing, and expressing thoughts and feelings through words and images and mental energies. Reiki is the spirit—the practice of channeling universal energy via a three-part connection from something greater than you (God, universe), through you (healer), and into someone you connect with who needs healing and balance (which could also be you).

But you probably already have some rituals you practice without realizing that's what they are. Do you check your phone every morning as soon as you wake up? That's a ritual. It might not be a ritual in the service of your highest good, but it's still a ritual. Do you always brush your teeth before you go to bed? That's a ritual. Do you make your coffee the same way every morning, or take the same train to work? Do you always have lunch at the same time, or walk your dog every day after work, or do you always call your parents on a certain day of the week? Do you go to a religious service every week, or go to the grocery store every Sunday? Do you have a day where you always take some time to do something you love, like read a book or go for a walk? Whatever it might be, those are all rituals.

Holidays are more obvious rituals. Are there certain things you always do on certain holidays, like visit family or bring out certain decorations year after year? Do you drink champagne at midnight on New Year's Eve? I have a friend who always makes sure that on *her* birthday, she sends her mother flowers, because, after all, her mother was the one who brought her into the world. Something I have always done, growing up in a Catholic household, where we did a traditional grace and blessing before meals, is to ritualize eating. What I do now is place my hands above my food and imagine healing and nourishment going into the food before I eat. If I choose to eat meat or fish, I also thank the animal it came from, and thank it for the experience of its life and for giving me nourishment and strength.

No matter what you already do, you can perform your rituals with more awareness and intention, and you can add rituals to all the parts of your life, wherever you feel you want or need them. In the next three chapters, I'm going to give you many of the rituals I do, along with many practices and exercises that can help you with your health and grounding, mind and purpose, energy and connection. Any practice can become a ritual, like walking barefoot in the grass on a warm day, or journaling every morning, or meditating every evening. Remember when you assessed which part of your triad of wholeness needed attention using the symptom lists in chapter 4? These rituals will help bring balance where you need it.

As you read through these next three chapters, stay open to what catches your attention. What sparks your interest? What sounds fun or fascinating or illuminating or necessary to you? Those are the rituals and practices to start with. Not everything in this book will be for you, and that's okay. But as much as you are willing to be open to the ideas and tools in this book, whatever it is you are seeking will come out and catch your attention. The more you stay open and curious about trying new things, the more you will find help and support for the direction in which you want to go. Even as someone who has been doing this work for more than a decade, I am still learning and I find there are still things that are new that I am skeptical of, until I realize that if I'm open, they might offer me something valuable. The more open you are, the more you will notice beautiful synchronicities that point you in the right direction.

To see how any of these practices, exercises, and rituals affect you, write about them in your journal and notice if anything changes. I've had many students come to me and say that even one week of ritualizing makes a difference. They say things like "Kelsey, just a week ago when I was writing in my journal, I was feeling overwhelmed and stressed, and everything seemed so hard! And today, after a week of ritualizing, I feel completely different!" Some of the rituals my students say work for them are blessing their food before eating it, doing a body check-in every day in the morning or in the middle of the day, journaling in the evening, having a cup of tea before bed, doing self-Reiki every day, setting intentions for the day, or creating a mental hygiene practice. Whatever you choose to start with, see how it changes how you feel after just seven days.

Rituals recognize that you are having this incredible one-of-a-kind life journey, so that you can switch off that autopilot that runs you through the same loop every day, as if it were always the same, without awareness of how each day is special. Rituals make being alive as a human on this earth feel miraculous. They make every experience feel important. What one person might see as mundane, what one person might not appreciate, another person can get joy and excitement and gratitude from by ritualizing it.

Let's get started with rock rituals that honor our body, our health, and the earth we stand on; the planets above us; and the cycles of nature.

~~~~~~

MORNING RITUAL

As I shared before, I never get out of bed, no matter how early I have to wake up or how late I might be for a meeting, without setting an intention or a prayer for myself for the day. When you clear your mind at the dawn of the day and set an intention for how you want the day to go, it helps to shift and clear any negative or cluttered morning vibes. Begin your day with a calm center and you can carry that calm throughout your day. Morning rituals can transition you from sleep to an expectant positive energy that prepares your body and mind for all the things you do. Here are some things to include in your morning ritual. Try some or all of these tomorrow morning:

- As soon as you wake up, even before you sit up, place your hands on your heart and take a few deep breaths.

- Keeping your hands over your heart, think of three things you are grateful for (no matter what you are feeling when you wake up).

- With your hands still on your heart, begin feeling your heartbeat and the breath flowing through your body. See yourself receiving love, health, and abundance throughout the day.

- Scan your body, starting at your toes and noticing how each part of you feels. Do you detect tightness, pain, tension, ease, relaxation, good feelings anywhere? Move from your feet up your legs, hips, stomach, chest, shoulders, arms, hands, neck, head. Whenever you sense pain or tension, imagine filling up that part of you with the energy of healing and love.

- When you feel relaxed, sit up in your bed slowly, and place your hands on your legs or in a prayer position in front of your heart.

- Begin to visualize how you'd like to see yourself throughout the day.

- Ask for guidance, support, and anything else you feel you are open to receiving. I like to end by using the prayer from *A Course in Miracles,* by Dr. Helen Schucman: *What would You have me do? Where would You have me go? What would You have me say, and to whom?* (In chapter 6, I mentioned this prayer.) You can use this or any other prayer that helps you set out with a feeling of purposefulness and direction.

~~~~~

A SIMPLE SELF-CARE TEA CEREMONY

A tea ceremony is a nice way to come back to center in the afternoon. Take a few minutes to boil some water and make yourself a cup of tea without rushing. Give the preparation process all your attention, as if it were a meditation. Use your own fresh herbs or any tea you like, but prepare it with care and a sense of nurturing yourself and giving yourself time to focus. Sit down and sip the tea and ask yourself, "How am I feeling right now?" Let yourself relax into your own space for just a little while before you rush off to finish your day. There are lots of great teas to calm the central nervous system, so perhaps try a more relaxing afternoon tea rather than that caffeine pick-me-up. I love lemon balm, rose tea, and chamomile for calming; dandelion for digestion; nettle tea for immunity; and peppermint for a nice soothing tea or post-big-afternoon meal.

~~~~~

EVENING RITUAL

You can piece together an evening ritual out of the things that you feel are helpful and enjoyable. What matters more than what you do is that you do it regularly, so your body learns that your ritual is a cue for sleep, and to include the element of slowing down and giving yourself permission to transition into nighttime. Day energy, like the energy from the sun, is bright and active, but night energy, like the energy from the moon, is cool and calm. Here are some things you can include in your evening ritual:

- Turn off all electronics, including your television and your phone, at least one hour before you want to be asleep. If you can, dim the lights in your home.

- Ritualize getting ready for tomorrow. Set out your clothes, make your lunch, make a list of the things you have to do tomorrow so you can get them out of your head.

- Journal. Lie in bed and write out a few things in your journal that you are grateful for. Or, if you tend to need more to calm down your busy and active mind, you could spend more time writing out all the different things that you are grateful for being able to accomplish in the day, and five or six things that you know you want to get accomplished in the next day. You could write about what you did that day that you are proud of, looking at yourself in a loving way. You could write what you could have done to be kinder to yourself that day. Then you can release that energy of the mind from needing to think and do.

- Do a few yoga poses to help your body slow down and to help your mind surrender. My favorite is to lie in child's pose for five minutes to empty out the day's energy from my entire body. Kneel on the floor with your knees apart, feet together, and bend forward, stretching your arms out in front of you, so you are resting your arms and forehead on the floor in a way that feels very comfortable, like you could fall asleep that way. (Use pillows to support you wherever you may need it, if necessary.)

- Make a cup of herbal tea and sip it slowly while reading a book or listening to calming music.

- Wipe the energy of the day off your body with little swipes of your hands all over yourself. Let yourself feel a sense of releasing everything you have had to carry with you throughout the day. You can also do this when you take a shower or a bath.

- Meditate, sitting in bed for about ten minutes, breathing and calming yourself down as you tell yourself that it's time for bed. You can tell yourself, "Thank you. You've done enough today," to transition into sleep mode.

- Right before sleep, lie in bed with your hands over your heart and reiki yourself to transition into sleep mode. (See page 234 for instructions on how to reiki yourself.)

BATHING RITUAL

Whenever I take a bath, I make it into a ritual. I make my bath so delicious—I light candles, I might prepare a cup of tea or eat a cookie, and I might play my favorite music. As I get into the bath, I think about giving myself permission to release the things that are not serving me. I take as long as I need, and when I'm done, as the bath drains, I watch all the unserving thoughts and energy I don't need going down the drain with the water, where it will dissipate harmlessly.

After a bath, you can also use a cream, oil, or lotion you love and take time to slowly massage it into your skin. As you do this, see yourself in full and complete health and vibrancy. I do this at night with arnica or CBD oil or essential oils. I rub them on my feet and thank my feet for all the places they carried me that day. I usually end by putting some rose oil on my chest over my heart as I imagine opening to love and to accepting more love.

RITUAL FOR MANIFESTING ABUNDANCE

One of the things that stresses people the most is money. If you wish for more resources to give you more freedom or less fear about not having a secure existence, try this ritual for abundance. This is a good ritual to do with a couple of friends who also feel that they need more abundance in their lives. I've done this with some of my girlfriends and we all love it and get to watch, in awe, what manifests.

Have each person doing the ritual bring a tall green candle (green represents money), a piece of paper, a pen, and a green crystal (like aventurine) to the ritual. Put the candle into a bowl and light it.

Position the crystals around the bowl. Sit in a circle around the candle, or face-to-face with the candle between you, if there are just two of you.

Taking turns, have each of you begin by sharing your gratitude for the abundance you already have in your life, whether that is material abundance, an abundance of health, an abundance of friends and family, an abundance of support, an abundance of professional opportunities, or whatever is true for you. Then, each of you shares what specific kind of abundance you would like to call into your life, such as money to afford a down payment on a new house, or money to pay off debts, or a greater or more reliable source of regular income, or even something less material, like an abundance of creativity or an abundance of wisdom.

Next, each of you answers three questions out loud to one another:

1. *What do you think is keeping you from receiving the abundance you desire?*

2. *What scares you about receiving the abundance you desire?*

3. *Why do you believe you can't have the abundance you desire?*

Whatever comes up—imprints, fear, energy blocks—give each other the permission to question the truth of those obstacles. Next, each of you writes down your prayer or wish for the abundance you desire on the piece of paper. Try to make these wishes very specific, such as how much money you want to see in your bank account or exactly how much money you want to have each month—even if it sounds unrealistic. Fold up the papers and put them in the bowl. Put the bowl in a safe place and let the candle burn all the way down, even if that takes a day. All the energy from the candle has to come all the way down to meet the wishes, infusing them with energy.

After your candle has burned down, take your crystal back and say: *I expect lavish abundance every day in every way in my life and affairs. I give incredible thanks for the lavish abundance I already possess today.*

Finally, for ten days, carry the crystal with you everywhere you go and repeat the above words once a day. Important: The moment you finish the chant each day, consciously let go of all expectation of a specific result. You have put the energy out there, so surrender and let the universe take over.

~~~~~~

RITUAL FOR HONORING YOURSELF

When you feel depleted or unappreciated, or when you can't see the big picture of your life and you feel that you haven't accomplished enough, try this meditation for honoring yourself and recognizing all your triumphs in your life journey so far. There is an apt Derren Brown quote I like to tell people before we do this meditation: "He who is not satisfied with the little is satisfied with nothing." When I do this as a guided meditation in my workshops, people often cry deeply, feeling the gratitude of their life in a new way.

Find a comfortable seated position. Close your eyes and take a few long, deep breaths, until you feel a sense of calm and peace within. Now slowly scroll backward in your mind through your life, all the way back to your earliest memories.

See yourself as a child. Try to remember something you did when you were very young. Gaze at that little child with fondness and compassion. See how beautiful, how innocent that child is? Fill your heart with love for that child's upcoming journey through life, which will be so full of wonder and learning. Take some time here.

Now think of yourself in those preteen years. Remember how you sometimes felt awkward or unsure, how much you wanted to fit in. Recall something you did that you always remembered as a good time, like a family trip or a fun day with your friends or a triumph in school. Think about what you were proud of, and send out compassion for all the things you felt insecure or afraid about. Send out love and appreciation to your younger self for making it through that difficult stage of growth. Stay here as long as you need to.

Now see yourself in high school, learning how to be an adult, step by step. Remember some of your most cherished friendships. Think about the challenges you faced. Think about your passions and the things that sparked your curiosity. Think about the dreams you had for your future, and send out so much love to that young adult you were becoming, despite your pain and sadness and difficulties. Think how much you endured, but kept going, kept living, kept surviving and hoping for the future. Take time to really inhabit this stage of your life in your memory and bless yourself with love and solidarity.

Now see yourself five years ago. Think about how old you were then. Think about how much you had learned by then, how much your childhood has stayed with you deep inside, what dreams you fulfilled, and what you were disappointed about. Think about what you were doing at that time in your life, and send out love to yourself for trying so hard, for enduring the frustration, for finding joy in life whenever you could, for continuing to search for your path.

Now count down the years—four years ago, three, two, one, spending as much time as you need to at each year of your life until you arrive back to your present self. How amazing you are! What an incredible journey it has been! Look back again over the arc of your life so far, as one long and incredible journey of life—the pain, the joy, the sadness, the challenges, the triumphs, the disappointments, the will you had to endure, the passions you chased, the loneliness, the connection, the emptiness, the fullness. See what a beautiful and complex person you have become? See what you have made it through? Send yourself love and honor yourself and your very human journey through all these years. Just keep sending love to yourself until you feel filled up with it.

When you are ready, slowly open your eyes. See if you can carry that love with you through the rest of your day, and week, and notice how it feels to truly honor yourself.

~~~~~

RITUAL FOR TRAVEL

I once experienced a terrifying emergency landing on a flight, so now I always ritualize any travel before I leave, whether it's in a plane or a car. Before I drive, I say a prayer. If you follow any particular religion, you can do a blessing or a prayer for the car. If you want to use elements of Reiki, you can lift up your hands and visualize energy from your body moving out through your hands and into the whole car, surrounding it with a shield of light and protection before you go out into the world.

Whenever I fly, as soon as I get on the plane, I'll lift my hands in front of my chest with my palms facing out, and I'll visualize the whole plane being bathed in light and protection. I send clarity and focus to the pilots. It's important to note that this is not to manipulate the energy of others. It's simply a way of putting a blessing onto the plane, the people on the plane, the flight, and the path of the flight. I visualize us getting to our destination safely and easily. Then I let go of any outcome. I have put my intention out there that we all have a safe and easy journey and that we get to our destination with ease and grace, but I also know that whatever happens and whatever comes up is meant to be. Because I always have a little bit of fear when it comes to flying, this is a great opportunity to give myself permission to surrender to the experience of the flight.

RITUAL FOR MOVING INTO A NEW SPACE

When my husband and I moved into our first new home together, it was really important to me that we put our energy and intentions into the space together so that it had both of our energies and desires, as individuals and as a couple. The day before the contractors put in the floors, we sat at the front door of the house and lit a candle I had purchased for home blessings. We had some incense, some sage, and a statue of Ganesh, the Hindu elephant god. My husband's family is Indian and his mother gave us this beautiful bronze statue for our home because Ganesh is the god of new beginnings.

What we did wasn't so much about the candle or the statue, but more about the lighting of our intentions together and the two of us coming together to honor the sacredness of our new home and the energy we were bringing into it. We sat there on the floor with our legs crossed, holding hands, and took some deep breaths together and started to think about how we wanted to see ourselves living in this home together with our two sons. We then shared those intentions with each other out loud and shared our gratitude. We thanked the home for taking us all in. We then wrote down our words on the concrete floor in fun-colored markers to bless the home with those desires. Then we went into the other rooms in the house and wrote down our intentions and words on the floors of those areas. For example, in the kitchen we wrote "health, laughter, happiness, togetherness, joy." In my office I wrote "clarity, abundance, integrity, joy, ease," and other words that felt aligned with my work. We knew the new floor would cover our colorful words. Now, even though we can't see them anymore, we know our words are under there, continuing to bless us and our home life together.

If you are moving into a new space, you could do what we did—although if you aren't getting new floors, you might not want to write all over them! Light a candle, thank the house, and set your intentions for the space and your future life there, preferably with everyone who will be living in the house. If you don't have the opportunity to write on a wall or a floor to embed your intentions and gratitude into the home, try lighting a candle and then making a list of all the things you *would* write. Place it somewhere special and tucked away for the home to receive—in a nook, under a floorboard, in the back of a cupboard—or ask the house where you should put it and see if you feel led somewhere. You are sharing your energy, intentions, and love with your new space so it can love and hold and support you in return.

HOME DETOX RITUAL

How do you feel when you walk in the door of your home or any room in your life? How does your body feel when you are in that place—your home in general, or a specific room, like your bedroom or kitchen? Do you feel energized and open in that space, or do you feel heavy, cluttered, and depleted? Clearing the space around your body can help make you feel lighter, more at ease, and open to whatever happens to you during your day. I do this in my own home regularly and I recommend doing it on some cyclical basis, whether it's daily, weekly, monthly, or seasonally, in order to shift and uplift the energy in the space where you spend so much of your time. Fire energy is especially powerful for cleansing the spaces in your life. You might try what I consider to be a house detox.

Get some sage or a clearing element like tuning forks, singing bowls, chimes, or a detox mist/spray. Hold it in your hand and walk around the room or the house, in the area you want to clear. Imagine dissolving the negative energy and the heavy vibrations you feel. Speak to your house and tell it you no longer need that negative energy and that you seek the highest good for your living space. Once you've walked through the space, thank the space for protecting and guiding you, and ask for its help in moving the negative energy out. Then, set an intention for the positive energy you want to bring into your new cleared space.

Now, if using sage, light it. The bundle should burn slowly and release smoke. Walk back through the space again, moving the plant through the room, into the corners, and wherever you feel that the energy might be "stuck." As you do this, ask the space to help you remove and release any energy that does not serve your highest good. When you feel that the room is cleansed, snuff out the fire. I like to then light incense and imagine that the incense smoke contains positive intentions for my space, coming in and infusing my home with the good energy I'm seeking.

If you're using sound clearing or a mist or spray, follow the same ritual, but either activate the sounds or spray the mist through the rooms, into the corners, and into the stuck places. I will often also open up the windows and doors to fully clear out and release the energy.

~~~~~

FOREST BATHING RITUAL

Forest bathing, or *shinrin-yoku*, is a therapeutic Japanese practice developed in the 1980s for taking in the medicine of the trees. All you do is walk through wooded areas with a lot of trees around you, but there are over one hundred scientific papers on the health benefits of forest bathing, or just spending time in nature with a lot of trees around. The biggest benefit seems to be for stress reduction.[1]

I was recently in France, where I participated in a two-hour walk through a forest that was designed specifically for forest bathing, along with interactive experiences and meditation chairs. One of the most significant things I learned from this experience is how important it is to disconnect from technology. Even if you bring a phone for safety reasons, it's important to put it away and resist the urge to take it back out and check it. If you feel compelled to take a picture or a video, don't do it. Instead, go out with the intention to explore and play and be bathed in nature. If you truly resist interacting with any technology, you will discover that you come out of your walk more alert, more awakened, and with a greater sense of clarity. It's a powerful experience.

There are many theories as to why forest bathing has such a positive effect. Just as the earth has electromagnetic energy to give us, trees have aromatic compounds (phytoncides) they release into the air, so when you walk through the forest, you are exposed to them. This is reported to boost immunity and increase natural killer cells, with effects that can last for a month after a single walk.

Some people theorize that it is just exposure to nature that is so healing, improving heart function and triggering parasympathetic instead of sympathetic nervous system activity.[2] One study showed that just looking at a house plant could increase levels of blood oxygen in the brain![3] Whatever the science behind it, it has been proven that walking through the woods reduces stress and improves health. Forest bathing takes only a little more effort than earthing—you just have to get to an area with a lot of trees. But whenever you get the chance, take a walk among the trees. Turn off your phone and go commune with nature. It's more earth medicine out there, waiting for you to take it in.

~~~

CHAPTER NINE

Paper: Rituals for the Mind

*Rituals are the formulas by which
harmony is restored.*

—TERRY TEMPEST WILLIAMS, AMERICAN WRITER AND CONSERVATIONIST

NEXT, LET'S MOVE to paper rituals that honor the mind, thoughts, feelings, planning, and life purpose. I hope you've already tried many of the exercises and journaling prompts earlier in the book, but if you are ready to go further, here are some rituals to calm, refine, sharpen, energize, and elevate your mind.

~~~

ANXIETY DIFFUSION RITUAL

Whenever you feel anxiety coming into your mind, try this ritual to support yourself in relieving the intensity.

- Sit comfortably and get quiet. Take a few conscious breaths. As you breathe in, notice the quality of your breath. Is it smooth, shaky, broken, shallow, deep? As you exhale, take it slow and make it last.

- Begin to count: Inhale for a slow count of four, and exhale for a slow count of eight. Do this ten times.

- Say to yourself, out loud or in your mind: "I am safe and all I need to do right now is breathe." Continue to breathe as you try to notice where in your body you feel the anxiety.

- Keep breathing in for four counts, out for eight counts.

- Place your hands on your heart and begin to send your breath to your heart space. Feel it expanding and filling with calm and peace.

- Keep repeating, "I am safe and all I need to do right now is breathe," until you feel a sense of calm come through your body.

- Keep doing this until you feel the anxiety start to subside. Slowly and calmly reenter your day.

~~~~

THE PENDULUM RITUAL

A pendulum is a fun tool for helping you externalize your internal voice, desires, and knowing. Pendulums can give you an answer about something you know on the inside when you can't access the information consciously—but, remember, the pendulum is accessing your inner wisdom, not some external all-knowing force. It doesn't predict some externally determined future. It is simply an intuition-accessing tool, so it meets you right where you are in the present moment. The answer may not be set in stone. If you ask a big question, like "Will I ever get married?," a pendulum might tell you yes on a Tuesday, but no on a Wednesday. That's because your path is never set and everything you do at any given moment determines your path. Where you are headed on a Tuesday might be different from where you are headed on a Wednesday.

You can buy a pendulum, which is often a crystal or another stone on a chain or cord, or you can make your own, using any weight on any kind of string. A pendant you wear as a necklace can also work.

To use a pendulum, put your elbow on a steady surface and hold the pendulum with your dominant hand, so the weight hangs straight down. If you don't have a steady surface, you can hold the top of the pendulum with your dominant hand and then place your nondominant hand in front of your stomach, palm up. Let the pendulum dangle just a couple of inches above your nondominant palm.

Begin by asking, "Show me my yes." Hold your dominant hand still and wait for the pendulum to move. It might swing backward and forward, side to side, or in a clockwise or counterclockwise circle. Whatever it does, that is your yes answer. Then ask, "Show me my no." The pendulum will make a different movement. Now you are ready to ask your question. The pendulum will answer you with a yes or no, as it was shown to you.

Sometimes I use my body like a pendulum, especially if I want to know if a particular supplement, medicine, or food is right for me at that moment. For example, I may want to know if a certain herb will be good for me. I will hold the herb, the capsules, or the bottle in my hands, close to my heart. Then I say to my body, "If this is a yes, let me move toward it. If this is a no, help me move away from it." Then I get quiet and just let the energy flow. My body will literally sway for a minute; then it will end up either moving forward or pulling away.

Sometimes I'll test it a couple of times just to get the rhythm and make sure I've got the right message, as my intuition speaks to me through my body. Anyone can do this. It's kind of fun, and an interesting way to work with your intuition and your body, to test something you want to try, especially once you begin trying a lot of different techniques and healing modalities, and reading about different herbs and food remedies. Nothing is right for everyone, so tapping into your intuition can help you figure out if something is right for you. The more you practice, even if it seems silly or odd at first, the more you strengthen your connection to your inner guidance and knowing.

~~~~~~

RITUAL FOR THE NEW MOON

Of all the planetary rituals (new moon, full moon, solstices, equinoxes), the new moon ritual is my favorite. To me, the new moon is like a blank canvas in the sky, onto which you can paint your intentions for faith, intuition, health, emotion, creativity, desire, and passion. Imagine that you are the most amazing painter—what are you going to put on that canvas for the upcoming month?

On the day of the new moon, begin thinking about all the things you seek to bring into your life related to intuition, emotion, and creativity. Think about the things you are passionate about and make you feel most like yourself, especially things you want to create. Envision the sky as an actual canvas, there above you in its new moon darkness, and picture what you would paint on it. What words, or images, or places, or moments do you see for yourself on that canvas? What energy will you put up there so it can come back and find you? Know that new moon energy is present twenty-four hours before and after the actual peak of the new moon, so you have a forty-eight-hour window to do this ritual. Here is an example of how I do a new moon ritual:

1. *I like to prepare for this ritual by taking a bath. Fill the bath with Dead Sea salt crystals or Epsom salts. Spend twenty to*

thirty minutes soaking in the bath. You are cleansing yourself to receive. Dry off and, maintaining a calm and quiet inner state, gather two pieces of paper, a pen, a dark blue candle, and a smoky quartz or other night-colored crystal.

2. *If you can, step outside for a few minutes to observe the night sky at its darkest, and the new moon, if you can see it. Set an intention for your ritual. Say out loud or to yourself: "I will discover what I am led to create during this next moon cycle."*

3. *Put on some calming, instrumental music and sit comfortably (inside or outside) in a quiet, clean place. Put the candle and the crystal in front of you. Light the candle. Close your eyes; take some slow, deep breaths; and imagine clearing and cleansing your mind and the space around you of any residue, heaviness, or negative energy.*

4. *Set an intention in your mind that this ritual will bring you inspiration for the month ahead. Visualize the dark sky of the new moon and think about how the moon is about to begin waxing and moving toward fullness from this empty space of potential. Meditate on this for five to ten minutes.*

5. *On the first piece of paper, write down how you have been feeling in the past month, both positive and negative. What has been going on in your life? Especially note any gratitude you are feeling for the past month.*

6. *On the second piece of paper, record the date, and write everything you intend and desire to bring into your life during this coming moon cycle. Be specific. What do you want to learn? How do you want to feel? What do you want to receive in your life? These should be things that, when you think of them, make you feel excited, alive, open, healthy, loved, balanced,*

connected, and joyful. Don't worry about how these things will come to you. Just list what you are ready to receive.

7. *Fold both pieces of paper. One at a time, place your hands over the papers. Bless the first sheet of paper for giving you the gift of experience and knowledge. Bless the second one for giving you the gift of hope and rekindled passion.*

8. *Put the pieces of paper and the crystal together, with the crystal on top of the folded papers, under your bed or under your mattress or on your altar or in any other sacred space. Leave it there until the next new moon, releasing any expectation of the result but allowing your intention to paint the canvas of the dark sky with your desires and the energy of your willingness to receive.*

RITUAL FOR THE FULL MOON

The full moon emits the most light when its energy is at its peak. On this day (or within a forty-eight-hour window), you are filled up with all the energy, thoughts, feelings, blessings, and challenges of the last month. Now the moon is about to wane, releasing its light, and this ritual is about releasing what no longer serves you so you can shift in new directions that are more in line with your current vibration and make room for new energies and opportunities that will keep you moving in the direction in which you want to go. Here's how I like to do it:

1. *Light some incense or sage, or use an energy-clearing mist. Clear the room where you are doing the ritual by moving through the room, clearing as you go with whatever method you choose.*

2. *Get a piece of paper, a pen, a candle, a clear or milky quartz crystal or other white or clear crystal, and a fire-safe bowl or can or a paper shredder.*

3. *Sit comfortably in a quiet, clean place. Put the candle and the crystal in front of you. Light the candle. Close your eyes; take some slow, deep breaths; and imagine your mind filled with the bright light of the full moon and all you have received over the past month. Meditate on this for five to ten minutes.*

4. *At the top of the paper, write "My Full Moon Release List." Make a list of all the things you intend to release, that have perhaps been helpful or harmful to you in the last month and that are no longer serving you and your highest good. What are you ready to let go of?*

5. *Read the list out loud or just to yourself and think about your readiness to really release these things from your life, then place your hands over the list and thank it for all you have learned and received.*

6. *Tear up the paper into pieces and put it in the fire-safe container. Set it on fire and watch it burn (or put it in the paper shredder). As you do this, imagine the energies from the things on your list dissolving with love and grace and dissipating into the atmosphere. To yourself or out loud, say: "I now willingly release these experiences, insecurities, fears, and pain. I let it all go with ease and grace. And so it is so."*

7. *Blow out the candle and discard the ashes or empty the shredder into the trash and take it outside. If you can see it, spend some time out there gazing at the full moon. Spend the rest of the evening thinking about who you can be now without those things you have set free.*

RITUAL FOR THE FIRST OF THE MONTH

With each new month, I always do a ritual to prepare for what is coming. This is a way of organizing my plans and intentions for the next month, so they are clear in my mind and present in my thoughts. I also do my own version of an old British tradition. Here's what I do:

ON THE LAST DAY OF THE PREVIOUS MONTH: In my journal, I write out all the things that I am grateful for that happened in that previous month.

ON THE FIRST DAY OF THE NEXT MONTH: First thing in the morning, I yell out, "White rabbit, white rabbit, white rabbit!" (My husband thinks I'm crazy, but this is an old tradition, thought to bring abundance to a new month or year—I think it is traditionally used on New Year's Day, but I like to do it monthly.) Then in my journal, I write out all the practical things I want to call into my life that month, such as meet a deadline, make contact with a friend, finish cleaning out a part of your home, or take a step toward a new goal.

At the top of the list, I put three things I am willing to actively do to create and manifest those things in my life. It might be something like "I willingly choose to make my doctor's appointment, book my trip for this summer, and reach out to those four people who have offered to help me get my website started." This makes the ritual not just about my intentions for the month, but about the active things I will do to make them happen in my life.

PRAYER BEFORE AN IMPORTANT
EVENT

When something big is happening that requires you to speak, make a presentation, convince others of a proposal or plan you created, or agree to something important, whether it's making a critical phone call, delivering a speech, negotiating a contract, running a meeting, taking a test, or having an emotionally charged conversation, this short prayer to your higher power, however you envision that, can help put your mind in the right place and help the right words to come through you:

I trust that I am enough. I trust that I am worthy. I trust that I have beautiful things to express. I trust that I will be guided in expressing those things with love, for the highest good of all. Let my thoughts be thoughts of love. Let my words be words of love. Let me remember that my love is enough.

CHAPTER TEN

Reiki: Rituals for the Spirit

Life is a verb, not a noun.

—CHARLOTTE PERKINS GILMAN, AMERICAN NOVELIST

THIS LAST CHAPTER of rituals focuses on energy. Every ritual and exercise here has to do with moving, shifting, increasing, or cleansing energy. My primary focus here is on Reiki, and on pages 230–240, you can find instructions for how to channel Reiki energy for healing yourself and others. But in this chapter, I include a simple version for simply feeling the energy.

HANDWASHING RITUAL

If you've been in meetings all day or around a lot of people, you can clear your energy, lift your spirits, and increase your good vibrations by consciously cleansing your hands. Go to the sink and take a moment to see your hands. Think about how they have literally been outwardly extending your energy into the world.

From handshakes to opening doors to sending emails to using cellphones or gesticulating to help get your point across to other people, your hands spend all day exchanging, giving, receiving, and connecting energies. Notice if they feel a little bit heavy.

Now turn on the faucet and allow cold water to pour down on your hands. Run the water over your wrists, your forearms, all the way up to your elbows. As the water goes up to the elbow on the first side, imagine that all the energy of your day that is connected to you is washing away down the drain. Repeat on the other side. Sweep the water off your arms with your hands.

Now check in with your hands again. Have you washed away the day's energy or perhaps the chaos or stress you may have felt? Do your hands feel as if they have released something? Do they feel lighter? Do they feel ready to receive and exchange new energy? If not, wash your hands again, and brush the water down your arms and off your fingertips. As you dry your hands and arms, thank the energy for exiting and see your arms filling up with light, space, openness, and new energy. After a day with lots of interactions or a lot of giving away of energy, this exercise is a great way to get back to yourself by restoring calm, clean energy to your hands that is just for you.

RITUAL FOR FEELING YOUR ENERGY

Every one of us has energy within us and around us and moving in and out of us, but because you can't feel it, it may not feel real. However, you actually *can* feel it. Try this exercise to physically feel the energy that can radiate from your palms, which is the energy you use when you practice Reiki.

- Sit comfortably, with a nice, upright posture, and close your eyes. Think about calming and softening your breath into a regular cadence with a balance of inhalation and exhalation. Take a few moments to get to this place of calm balance as you smooth the rhythm of your breath. If you need to do some open-mouth vocal exhalations to release any excess energy, you can do that, too.

- Let your hips begin to feel heavy, dropping into the earth. Let yourself be supported by the earth. Let yourself be held. Give yourself permission to let go of your own weight, and to let go of anything you believe you have to carry—thoughts, worries, or burdens. Let it all go.

- Begin to soften your muscles, and think about softening your tendons, ligaments, and fibers. Soften your bones. Soften your cells. Soften your thoughts. Give yourself permission to be right here, inside your body, right now.

- When you're ready, feel the crown of your head, and see if you can feel the space just a couple inches above the top of your head. Feel that space softly opening, the head softly opening.

- Allow healing, divine energy in the form of light coming in through that space and into the crown of your head. Feel it moving in a column of light down into your heart, then out into every cell of your body, from the center down your arms and legs, filling you with light.

- Now notice that with each inhalation, you draw more of this light energy in through your crown, and with each exhalation, you send that energy into every part of your body, lighting up every muscle, every fiber, every bone, every cell, and every thought. Inhale to receive, exhale to light up your cells and thoughts.

- When you're ready, gently lift your hands in front of your heart and hold them close together but not touching, as if you have a small ball in your hands. Relax your shoulders, your elbows, your fingers. Relax your jaw and neck. Keep the rhythm going, inhaling energy into the body, exhaling energy into every cell and every thought.

- Now begin to move your hands around, feeling that ball of energy in your palms. Move your hands slightly apart and slightly closer together. Play a little bit. See if you can feel the energy accumulating between your palm chakras. Don't worry if you don't feel what you think you will feel. Just play and keep your awareness open.

- When you feel that it's time to stop, gently place your hands onto your legs. Take a nice, big, deep inhale, then a big, open exhale. Inhale again, tucking your chin. Exhale again, opening your eyes.

Did you feel something between your palms? If you did, that, my dear, is Reiki energy. If you didn't, just keep practicing. The energy is there, whether you feel it or not, but the more you open your awareness and refine your sensitivity, the more easily you will be able to feel it.

~~~~~

CHAKRA BALANCING RITUAL

The chakras along the center of your body are energy centers and when energy is flowing through you, it can move through all the chakras, up and down your center, without any blocks. I do this meditation ritual as it was passed to me by my Reiki master and as I share it with my Reiki 1 students. I also use it whenever I feel that I need to clear out blockages in any of my chakras. Even if you aren't sure what might be blocked, you can use this ritual anytime you want to feel better, stronger, more healthful energy movement up and down, from the base of your spine (your first chakra) to the crown of your head (your seventh chakra).

- Sit comfortably in a chair with your feet flat on the ground, preferably barefoot. Take some calm, balanced breaths. Put your hands on your legs or in your lap.

- Visualize your feet rooting down into the earth. Feel your hands becoming heavy. Feel the heaviness in your knees and hips. Feel your entire being sinking and relaxing deeper and deeper into the weight and security of the planet.

- Let your shoulders soften. Relax your jaw. Relax your tongue. Let your shoulders drop down even farther from your ears.

- Find yourself right here in this moment, on this day, in this space, willing to be here, willing to connect to your own energy in a harmonious way.

- With every exhalation, release any anticipation, expectation, holding, carrying. Surrender to the here and now, letting this present moment be enough.

- Now begin to see yourself, dressed all in white, standing on a beach. The warm sun above, the water is cleansing and clearing, washing away any doubts, any heaviness, any pain. An energy of peace sweeps down through your entire body and you feel a deep sense of knowing that you are coming home to your true, divine, infinite self.

- Feel all the elements around you. Listen to the sound of the water. Feel the warmth of the sun. Smell the salt air. Feel your feet in the sand and the water.

- Look down the beach. You see a path leading up the beach toward a small opening in the rocks. Begin walking toward the path. Follow the path up to this small opening. As you get nearer, the opening grows bigger and you know this is a sacred space, meant for you to enter.

- Step toward the opening in the rocks. Turn back to take one more look at the beach and feel that sense of peace coming into your body again, then turn toward the cave.

- As you step inside, you see what looks like a beautiful, magical kingdom of crystals—there are crystals everywhere, sparkling and glinting. You know these crystals are healing crystals and they are there for you. You feel that they are almost smiling at you because you have finally made it back home to your sanctuary. Feel the healing and loving energy coming from the crystals. Open yourself to receiving it and knowing that everything here is just for you.

- Now you see that, in the center of this crystal cave, there's a staircase. You walk toward it and you see that there is a crystal embedded in each step. On the first step is a beautiful, deep red agate. You step up onto the first step and put both feet on this stone. You feel healing energy flowing up through your feet, up your legs, and into your root chakra at the base of your spine. You feel flooded with healing and a strong sense of safety and security.

- The next step contains a brilliant orange-colored citrine. You step onto it with both feet and you feel energy pouring into your feet and moving up your body, through your root chakra and into your sacral chakra, just below your navel. You feel it clearing, opening, and healing your organs, your digestive system, and your sense of inner knowing.

- The next step contains a third stone—a soft yellow quartz crystal. You step onto this stone and you feel the energy pouring up through your feet, through your root chakra, through your sacral chakra, and into your solar plexus, just below your rib cage. You feel a wave of emotional healing and a sense of peace and solace about everything you have ever experienced. You feel another wave of forgiveness washing over you.

- The next step contains a gorgeous, clear bright green emerald. Energy flows through your feet, up through your root chakra, your sacral chakra, and your solar plexus, then you feel a blast of love, like you've never known, pouring into your heart, opening, clearing, and moving the energy. You feel an overwhelming essence of unconditional love.

- The next step contains a deep blue lapis lazuli. As you step onto this stone, the energy moves through your feet, flowing upward through your root chakra, your sacral chakra, your solar plexus, through your heart and into your throat chakra. You feel a surge of opening, inner light, and a sense of understanding truth and the ability to communicate clearly, speaking your truth and expressing your needs without any hindrance or confusion. You feel an opening in your neck and throat and jaw.

- The next step contains a spectacular purple amethyst crystal. As you step onto it, you feel energy moving up through your feet into your root chakra, through your stomach and solar plexus, through your heart and throat, then deep, deep, deep into the center of your skull. You feel a deep sense of connection to infinite wisdom and you feel your third eye, in the center of your forehead, opening to see exactly who you are and who you came here to be. You have a vision of your life as easy, flowing, and living your truth.

- The last step contains a bright, majestic diamond. As you step onto this diamond, energy flows up through your feet, through your root, your stomach, your solar plexus, heart, throat, your third eye, and then up into the crown of your head. You feel the energy begin to surge, moving from your crown up far above you, and down, connecting your feet to the earth. It cycles up and down, from the center of the earth, through you, and back up to the sky, the stars. Feel that energy as it moves through you, as part of a chain of infinite moving energy. Just feel it and allow your body to receive it.

- Look straight up. Above you, the top of the cave slowly begins to open. You see the light of sun and stars and moon and sky, all at the same time. You have a sense of complete freedom, both grounded in what supports you and connected to what sends energy through you, fully integrated into the universe and healed by its light.

- Now you look back down the stairway and see the opening you came through. You turn and slowly walk back down the stairs, back down from the diamond to the amethyst, to the lapis lazuli, the emerald, the quartz, the citrine, and the agate, then back through the room of crystals. You step back out of the cave and back onto the beach.

- Begin to come back into your body. Place your hands in prayer position and, when you are ready, open your eyes.

CRYSTAL RITUALS

Crystals come from the earth and are literally rocks, but because they contain their own energy and healing vibrations, I consider them tools for spiritual healing more than for physical healing. If you are sensitive, you may be able to feel the energetic vibration of crystals when you hold them. Some people get visual images when they hold a crystal. Others feel an actual vibration, or heat or coolness coming from them.

The research behind crystals isn't exactly hard science, but that hasn't stopped people from collecting them, wearing them, placing them around their homes and offices, using Himalayan salt lamps and magnetic bracelets, and studying charts and books about what different crystals can do. Some scientists who are working outside the mainstream claim that they can measure the energy in crystals, that crystals are quantum converters that can transmit energy, rearrange and organize the molecular structure of water, and have biological effects on the human body.[1]

Personally, I think crystals are a wonderful way to start bringing the arts of metaphysics and energy healing into your home. One of the first things that attracted me to the world of energy healing was my love of crystals. I don't recall much about crystals from childhood, except for the family trips we took to the mining towns in the Midwest where we would pan for gold. We never found any gold, but we did find a lot of cool rocks and some crystals. I would collect them and hold them and play with them when I got back home.

As I got older, I began to associate crystals with "hippie" types of people and I didn't think that was me, so my interest waned. However, when I started getting into Reiki, I started to see more crystals around, since I was in more healing environments. As I gained sensitivity, I began to feel their energy. I noticed which ones I felt more connected to, and I would gravitate toward those. Now I keep them all over my home and use them often for grounding, peace, and healing.

Whether you can detect crystal energy or not, working with crystals can give you a sense of support from the earth and bring earth energy into your home and into your body. An easy way to begin is to visit a crystal shop and wander around. Just browse and see if you can feel the energy. Don't just grab the first ones you see. Take some time. Pick up different ones. See how they feel in your hands. Which ones attract you? Which ones feel as if they hum with energy? When you find one that speaks to you in some energetic way, that's the one you need. It's calling for you to take it home.

Many people say that certain crystals called out to them, and that is how they chose what to bring home. Every crystal has a different kind of energy and you can use different crystals for different purposes. I feel the energy of different crystals differently over time, but in the beginning, I remember there were three that I could not get enough of. These are the crystals I recommend for anyone who is just beginning to pay attention to energy, or who is just getting interested in crystals. These three make the perfect beginner's crystal starter kit. They connect to most of the things that people need when they first start to walk down a spiritual path:

- **QUARTZ CRYSTAL**: This is one of the master stones, known for its ability to bring clarity by releasing negative or unwanted energy, while also helping to amplify the energy in any space and to support manifesting your desires and healing you at every level. This is a good crystal to keep around your house, on your desk at work, or in any place where you want to release negative energy and have a clear mind.

- **ROSE QUARTZ**: This is the love stone. It is the perfect crystal for healing, for cultivating self-love, and for bringing a tremendous amount of compassion to the journey into the self. It can help you to feel more love and compassion for others and soften your view. Rose quartz is still my all-time favorite stone. This is a good crystal to keep beside your bed, or in a room where loved ones often gather. Or, if you work with clients, keep this one in your workspace, to be more compassionate in your interactions.

- **AMETHYST**: This is a powerful stone that supports spiritual balance and healing. It assists with intuition and sparks vivid dreams. It also helps to release anxiety and old, fixed, negative behaviors and habits. It is a spiritual cleanser and protector. When you feel that you need more vision, more connection to your inner knowledge, or more balance, call on amethyst. Amethyst is also a good crystal to keep by your bed if you want your dreams to be more intuitive, or keep it wherever you do any spiritual work, such as meditation, prayer, or energy healing.

Keep your stones in a clean, safe place, like a soft bag or a box you love, or put them in a place where you can see them and touch them frequently, like on your desk, beside your bed, or anywhere you need that crystal's particular energy and influence. Some people also like to carry small crystals in their pockets or in a small pouch they wear around their neck or waist. Some crystals are also included in powerful jewelry, as amulets, rings, or bracelets.

Wherever you keep your crystals, handle them. Hold them close to your heart for love (especially rose quartz), your solar plexus for courage (especially clear quartz), or your forehead ("third eye") for clear thinking (try amethyst here). Every crystal is a little different, so get to know yours and you'll get better at figuring out how crystals can help and heal you. You can incorporate your crystals into your meditations by holding them, or you can carry them with you when you need extra support. You can also include them when you do Reiki by putting them over the spot that needs energy while you also reiki that area.

✦ CHARGING YOUR ✦
CRYSTALS

Just as batteries occasionally need to be recharged, crystals you use frequently (or that you haven't used in a while) also need occasional recharging. An easy way to do this is to rinse your crystal in water to remove any dust or smudges, then set it out in the moonlight. The crystal should be in contact with the light for at least a few hours, preferably all night when the sky is clear and the moon is full. You can also charge your crystals by putting them next to a healthy plant or tree for a day or two, or by putting them in a bowl and covering them with salt or saltwater for up to twenty-four hours.

CHAPTER ELEVEN

Integration, and a Love Letter to Yourself

"What day is it?" asked Pooh.
"It's today," squeaked Piglet.
"My favorite day," said Pooh.

—A. A. MILNE, ENGLISH AUTHOR

EVERY DAY IS its own majesty. Every moment is its own creation. Life feels complex, but it is really very simple: Awareness without effort, acceptance without control, surrender without fear, and caring for yourself so you can show up for the world. There is a lot of material in this book—a lot of ideas, a lot of tools, a lot of resources for you, as you need them. You don't have to remember it all right now, but at the beginning of each day, or week, or month, or at any interval that makes the most sense and feels right to you, you can make a list of the things you want to accomplish during that period. I hope you will dip into this book frequently to find the tools that speak to you. Trust that when you are ready for them, they will catch your attention. Always put your own needs first—and once you have met your own needs, you will always know where you are needed. I believe we are all here to reach out and help each other, but helping others must come out of your own fullness. You can't help from a place of emptiness, burnout, and depletion.

Like me, you may always struggle a little bit with anxiety, stress, fear, sadness, or chronic pain. You may live with stress. But now you have the tools to manage it. Now you know how to become aware of it. Now you know how important it is to feel your feelings and let them pass, and to check in with your body, your mind, and your spirit every day, to be sure you are living the life you were put here to live with all the energy and passion you have inside you. Living is an art and it takes practice to do it well, but, within, you are a genius at living. Look within to access your own virtuosity.

If you like reminders, keep in mind these eleven basic things you can do to stay in health and awareness, and to cultivate inner calm and spaciousness in your life, no matter what happens to you:

1. *Create a morning ritual and an evening ritual for yourself. Commit to them.*

2. *Eat intuitively, move naturally, and honor your health.*

3. *Bring nature into your circle of awareness.*

4. *Check in with your energy every day and honor where you are at each moment.*

5. *Give yourself permission to do what brings you joy, to be who you are, and to live according to your own inner rhythms.*

6. *Find your purpose and own your power—and live your life accordingly.*

7. *Embrace change because change is inevitable.*

8. *Surrender control because control is an illusion.*

9. *Ritualize the moments, cycles, and events in your life, to honor the sacred nature of life.*

10. *Connect with yourself, with other beings, and with universal energy, and in every moment of your existence, you will continually feel your own becoming.*

11. *Be a light unto yourself, and you will be a light unto the world.*

I want to end this book with a love letter to you—it is from me to you, but I also want you to think of it as from you to you. Just as you read the agreement at the beginning of this book, I would love for you to read this letter out loud to yourself. Read it slowly and let the words sink into your heart, infusing your body, your mind, and your spirit with healing, loving, universal energy. Do your best to believe every word, because I promise you that every word of it is true. If it helps, read it to yourself often, and you may find that you believe it a little more each time. Here it is, just for you, and may your heart be filled with blessings and love today and always.

TO MY DEAREST, MOST BELOVED SELF:

You are a beautiful soul. Everything about you is beautiful. Every molecule within you is more precious than a diamond.

My wish for you is that you live in each present moment with awareness and surrender.

That you take responsibility for your own fullness so you can live with purpose and give without effort.

That you will always meet your own needs, so you can feel where you are needed.

That you recognize your supreme and absolute worthiness.

That you embrace a willingness to live in your fullness and incandescence.

That you find a way each day to step into your power.

That you will be willing to ask for help when you know you need it, even if it feels scary.

You are a force of nature. You are wholly and perfectly unique and there will never be anyone else like you in all time and in all the universe.

You are a channel for light. You are light.

You are love. You deserve love. It is your birthright!

You deserve health. You have a purpose. You are safe to connect.

You already have all these things within you.

You deserve to take the time and sacred resources to bring each one of these things to the surface and live them.

You deserve everything you desire.

You are worthy of a miraculous life.

You deserve to burn bright, and to cast your luminous brilliance out over the world, for your own highest good, and for the highest good of all beings.

I see you. I bow to you. I am you.

ACKNOWLEDGMENTS

First and foremost, thank you to Anna, Sarah, Celeste, and the Park-Fine literary team. You have believed in me and my ability to create this book since day one. I could not have gotten here without you.

To Eve, my amazing cowriter. What would I have done without you on this journey? Your patience, brilliance, dedication, and respect for the contents of these pages have given this book the energy, life, and professionalism it needed to be made manifest.

To the Harmony team, I am so honored to write my first book with all of you. Thank you for giving me the opportunity to share these teachings, practices, and rituals in a way that I would not have been able to do on my own or in person. I am so deeply humbled to be one of the Penguin Random House authors.

To Chris Richards, thank you for your time, energy, and incredible edits to this manuscript. You are a beloved and trusted friend.

To every single student, client, and teacher I have encountered along my path, thank you for standing side by side with me in this human journey. Each and every one of us is both a student and a teacher in this life. I bow to the teachers who have helped me get to this place in my life, and I bow to the clients and students who have given me a space to step into the teacher I have become today.

And to Arianna Huffington, a woman I deeply respect and admire, for creating the much-needed awareness around burnout. She is brightening the path for us all as she works to change the "collective delusion that burnout is the price we must pay for success."

To my nearest and dearest friends, because of your unconditional love and support, things like this book have become possible.

Having you by my side through the good times and the bad and sharing our spiritual practices and growth together have brought so much ease and grace into my day-to-day life. I can't wait to keep sharing this life with you and finding the joy throughout the journey.

To Mom, Dad, Cassie, and Mitch, I thank God every day for our family of five. So much of what I love in this life is because of the four of you. Thank you for loving me, for pushing me, laughing with me, dancing with me, and supporting me through all these years.

To Apurva, Devan, and Caden. You three men are my world. I love you and am so blessed to be loved by you.

Finally, I'd like to acknowledge all of the other human beings out there who are forging the path for a new way of living. It is not always easy to share new ideas, new ways of thinking, and new concepts to our mainstream society. May we continue to have the courage to support one another as we burn bright and light up the world with our love.

NOTES

CHAPTER 1: Awareness: The Age of Anxiety

1 National Institutes of Health, "5 Things You Should Know about Stress," https://www.nimh.nih.gov/health/publications/stress/index.shtml; American Psychological Association 2015 Stress in America Stress Snapshot, https://www.apa.org/news/press/releases/stress/2015/snapshot; Global Organization for Stress, www.gostress.com/stress-facts/; and Anxiety and Depression Association of America, https://adaa.org/understanding-anxiety/related-illnesses/stress. Some of this information was compiled in an online article called "23 Unnerving Stress Statistics" by Rebecca Lake, published on May 1, 2019, on the website CreditDonkey, https://www.creditdonkey.com/23-stress-statistics.html.

2 *One Nation under Stress*, documentary directed by Marc Levin, starring Dr. Sanjay Gupta, CNN chief medical correspondent, that debuted on HBO in 2019.

3 Jamie Ducharme, "More Than 90 percent of Generation Z Is Stressed Out," *Time* magazine, published online October 30, 2018, http://time.com/5437646/gen-z-stress-report/.

4 Cigna U.S. Loneliness Index, 2018, https://www.multivu.com/players/English/8294451-cigna-us-loneliness-survey/docs/IndexReport_1524069371598-173525450.pdf.

5 Asurion 2018 Consumer Tech Dependency Survey press release, https://www.asurion.com/about/press-releases/americans-equate-smartphone-access-to-food-and-water-in-terms-of-life-priorities/.

6 Adam Alter, *Irresistible: The Rise of Addictive Technology and the Business of Keeping Us Hooked* (New York: Penguin Press, 2017).

7 World Health Organization, "Burn-out an 'occupational phenomenon': International Classification of Diseases," Mental Health Home: https://www.who.int/mental_health/evidence/burn-out/en/.

8 Sighard Neckel, Anna Katharina Schaffner, and Greta Wagner, eds., *Burnout, Fatigue, Exhaustion: An Interdisciplinary Perspective on a Modern Affliction* (CITY: Palgrave Macmillan, 2017).

CHAPTER 2: Imprints: Your Pain Story

1 Rose McDermott, James Fowler, and Nicholas Christakis, "Breaking Up Is Hard to Do, Unless Everyone Else Is Doing It Too: Social Network Effects on Divorce in a Longitudinal Sample," *Social Forces* 92, no. 2 (2013): 491–519.

1 https://www.cdc.gov/chronicdisease /resources/press_room.htm.

2 https://www.aarda.org /news-information/statistics/.

3 https://www.cdc.gov/mmwr /volumes/66/wr/mm6645a1 .htm?s_cid=mm6645a1_w.

4 M. H. Christoph, K. A. Loth, M. E. Eisenberg, A. F. Haynos, N. Larson, and D. Neumark-Sztainer, "Nutrition Facts Use in Relation to Eating Behaviors and Healthy and Unhealthy Weight Control Behaviors," *Journal of Nutritional Education and Behavior* 50, no. 3 (2018): 267–274.

5 K. A. Romano, M. A. Swanbrow Becker, C. D. Colgary, and A. Magnuson, "Helpful or Harmful? The Comparative Value of Self-Weighing and Calorie Counting versus Intuitive Eating on the Eating Disorder Symptomology of College Students," *Eating and Weight Disorders: Studies on Anorexia, Bulimia and Obesity* 23, no. 6 (December 2018): 841–848.

6 J. M. Warren, N. Smith, and M. Ashwell, "A Structured Literature Review on the Role of Mindfulness, Mindful Eating and Intuitive Eating in Changing Eating Behaviors: Effectiveness and Associated Potential Mechanisms," *Nutrition Research Reviews* 30, no. 2 (December 2017): 272–283.

7 D. L. Rosenbaum and K. S. White, "The Role of Anxiety in Binge Eating Behavior: A Critical Examination of Theory and Empirical Literature," *Health Psychology Research* 1, no. 2 (April 2013): e19, https://www.ncbi.nlm .nih.gov/pmc/articles/PMC4768578/.

8 "Research Roundup: Benefits of Massage Therapy for Self-Care," American Massage Therapy Association. Online article with multiple research links: https://www.amtamassage.org /research/Massage-Therapy-Research -Roundup/Research-Roundup--Benefits -of-Massage-Therapy-for-Self-Care .html.

9 T. Williams, "CBD Is Wildly Popular: Disputes Over Its Legality Are a Growing Source of Tension," *New York Times,* published online May 6, 2019, https://www.nytimes.com/2019/05/06 /us/cbd-cannabis-marijuana-hemp .html.

10 University of East Anglia, "It's Official— Spending Time Outside Is Good for You," *Science Daily,* published online July 6, 2018, https://www.sciencedaily.com /releases/2018/07/180706102842.htm.

11 G. Chevalier, S. T. Sinatra, J. L. Oschman, K. Sokal, and P. Sokal, "Earthing: Health Implications of Reconnecting the Human Body to the Earth's Surface Electrons," *Journal of Environmental and Public Health* (2012), published online January 12, 2012, https://www.ncbi.nlm.nih.gov /pmc/articles/PMC3265077/.

12 J. L. Oschman, G. Chevalier, and R. Brown, "The Effects of Grounding (Earthing) on Inflammation, the Immune Response, Wound Healing, and Prevention and Treatment of Chronic Inflammatory and Autoimmune Diseases," *Journal of Inflammation Research* 8 (2015): 83–96. Published online March 24, 2015, https://www .ncbi.nlm.nih.gov/pmc/articles /PMC4378297/.

13 M. Ghaly and D. Teplitz, "The Biologic Effects of Grounding the Human Body during Sleep as Measured by Cortisol Levels and Subjective Reporting of Sleep, Pain, and Stress," *Journal of Alternative and Complementary Medicine* 10, no. 5 (October 2004): 767–776.

14 D. Brown, G. Chevalier, and M. Hill, "Pilot Study on the Effect of

Grounding on Delayed-Onset Muscle Soreness," *Journal of Alternative and Complementary Medicine* 16, no. 3 (March 2010): 265–273.

15 G. Chevalier, K. Mori, and J. L. Oschman, "The Effect of Earthing (Grounding) on Human Physiology," *European Biology and Bioelectromagnetics* 2, no. 1 (2006): 600–621.

16 G. Chevalier, "Changes in Pulse Rate, Respiratory Rate, Blood Oxygenation, Perfusion Index, Skin Conductance, and Their Variability Induced during and after Grounding Human Subjects for 40 Minutes," *Journal of Alternative and Complementary Medicine* 16, no 1 (January 2010): 81–87.

17 R. Klavinski, "7 Benefits of Eating Local Foods," Michigan State University Extension, published online April 13, 2013, https://www.canr.msu.edu /news/7_benefits_of_eating_local_foods.

18 L. Schiff and H. Kline, "Water's Wonders," *Psychology Today* (September 1, 2001), https://www .psychologytoday.com/us/articles /200109/waters-wonders.

19 A. Myles, "Scientific Facts That Make Me Want to Start Smudging Right Now," *Elephant Journal,* published online November 21, 2016, https://www .elephantjournal.com/2016/11/scientific -facts-that-make-me-want-to-start -smudging-right-now/.

20 C. S. Nautiyal, P. S. Chauhan, and Y. L. Nene, "Medicinal Smoke Reduces Airborne Bacteria," *Journal of Ethnopharmacology* 114, no. 3 (2007): 446–451, http://www.greenmedinfo .com/article/medicinal-smoke-can -completely-eliminate-diverse-plant -and-human-pathogenic-ba.

21 N. T. Tildesley, D. O. Kennedy, E. K. Perry, C. G. Ballard, S. Savelev, K. A. Wesnes, and A. B. Scholey, "*Salvia lavandulaefolia* (Spanish Sage) Enhances Memory in Healthy Young Volunteers," *Pharmacology Biochemistry and Behavior* 75 (2003): 669–674.

22 N. Abdi, "6 Benefits of Palo Santo," *Bodhi Tree Mind Body Soul,* published online October 16, 2018, https://bodhitree.com /journal/6-benefits-of-palo-santo/.

CHAPTER 6: The Burning Bright Mind

1 "Faith, Hope & Psychology, 80% of Thoughts Are Negative . . . 95% Are Repetitive," *The Miracle Zone: Practical Living in a Religious World,* published online March 2, 2012, https:// faithhopeandpsychology.wordpress .com/2012/03/02/80-of-thoughts-are -negative-95-are-repetitive/.

2 T. Newman, "Placebos: The Power of the Placebo Effect," *Medical News Today,* published online September 7, 2017, https://www.medicalnewstoday.com /articles/306437.php.

3 M. A. Piercy, J. J. Sramek, N. M. Kurtz, and N. R. Cutler, "Placebo Response in Anxiety Disorders," *Annals of Pharmacotherapy* 30, no. 9 (1996): 1013–1019.

4 R. Eccles, "The Powerful Placebo in Cough Studies?," *Pulmonary Pharmacology & Therapeutics* 15, no. 3 (2002): 303–308.

5 S. M. Patel, W. B. Stason, A. Legedza, S. M. Ock, T. J. Kaptchuk, L. Conboy, K. Canenguez, J. K. Park, E. Kelly, E. Jacobson, C. E. Kerr, and A. J. Lembo, "The Placebo Effect in Irritable Bowel Syndrome Trials: A Meta-Analysis," *Neurogastroenterology & Motility* 17, no. 3 (2005): 332–340.

6 T. J. Kaptchuk, E. Friedlander, J. M. Kelley, M. N. Sanchez, E. Kokkotou, J. P. Singer, M. Kowalczykowski, F. G. Miller, I. Kirsch, and A. J. Lembo, "Placebos without Deception: A Randomized Controlled Trial in Irritable Bowel Syndrome," *PLOS One* 5, no. 12 (2010): e15591, https://www.ncbi.nlm.nih.gov /pubmed/21203519.

7 American Psychological Association, "Multitasking: Switching Costs," published online March 20, 2006, https://www.apa.org/research/action /multitask.

8 E. Ophir, C. Nass, and A. D. Wagner, "Cognitive Control in Media Multitaskers," *Proceedings of the National Academy of Sciences of the United States of America (PNAS)* 106, no. 37 (2009): 15583–15587.

9 D. Bach, G. Groesbeck, P. Stapleton, R. Sims, K. Blickheuser, and D. Church, "Clinical EFT (Emotional Freedom Technique) Improves Multiple Physiological Markers of Health," *Journal of Evidence-Based Integrative Medicine* 24 (2019): 1–12.

CHAPTER 7: The Burning Bright Spirit

1 Emma M. Seppälä, "Connect to Thrive: Social Connection Improves Health, Well-Being, and Longevity," *Psychology Today*, published online August 26, 2012, https://www.psychologytoday .com/us/blog/feeling-it/201208/connect -thrive.

2 Maria Cohut, "What Are the Health Benefits of Being Social?," *MedicalNewsToday*, published online February 23, 2018, https://www .medicalnewstoday.com/articles/321019 .php.

3 Ana Sandoiu, "Having Close Friends May Stave Off Mental Decline," *MedicalNewsToday*, published online November 5, 2017, https://www .medicalnewstoday.com/articles/319978 .php.

4 Debra Umberson and Jennifer Karas Montez, "Social Relationships and Health: A Flashpoint for Health Policy," *Journal of Health and Social Behavior* 51 (Supplement) (2010): s54–66, https:// www.ncbi.nlm.nih.gov/pmc/articles /PMC3150158/.

5 Ibid.

6 Susan Pinker, "The Secret to Living Longer May Be Your Social Life," TED Talk 2017, https://www.ted.com /talks/susan_pinker_the_secret_to _living_longer_may_be_your_social _life?language=en.

7 Ibid.

8 Dan Buettner, *The Blue Zones: 9 Lessons for Living Longer from the People Who've Lived the Longest* (Washington, DC: National Geographic, 2008), https:// www.amazon.com/Blue-Zones-Second -Lessons-Longest/dp/1426209487.

9 Jeffrey M. Jones, "U.S. Church Membership Down Sharply in Past Two Decades," *Gallup Poll Social Series*, published online April 18, 2019, https:// news.gallup.com/poll/248837/church -membership-down-sharply-past-two -decades.aspx.

10 X. C. Ma, D. Jiang, W. H. Jiang, F. Wang, M. Jia, J. Wu, K. Hashimoto, Y. H. Dang, C. G. Gao, "Social Isolation–Induced Aggression Potentiates Anxiety and Depressive-Like Behavior in Male Mice Subjected to Unpredictable Chronic Mild Stress," *PLOS One* 6, no. 6 (2011): e20955: https://www.ncbi.nlm.nih .gov/pubmed/21698062; C. W. Fischer, N. Liebenberg, B. Elfving, S. Lund, and G. Wegener, "Isolation-Induced

Behavioral Changes in a Genetic Animal Model of Depression," *Behavioral Brain Research* 230, no. 1 (2012): 85–91.

11 Laurel Braitman, *Animal Madness: How Anxious Dogs, Compulsive Parrots, and Elephants in Recovery Help Us*

Understand Ourselves (New York: Simon & Schuster, 2014).

12 R. L. Zasloff and A. H. Kidd, "Loneliness and Pet Ownership among Single Women," *Psychological Reports* 75, no. 2 (1994): 747–752.

CHAPTER 8: Rock: Rituals for the Body

1 M. M. Hansen, R. Jones, and K. Tocchini, "Shinrin-Yoku (Forest Bathing) and Nature Therapy: A State-of-the-Art Review," *International Journal of Environmental Research and Public Health* 14, no. 8 (2017): 851, https://www.ncbi.nlm.nih.gov/pmc/articles/PMC5580555/.

2 C. Song, H. Ikei, and Y. Miyazaki, "Physiological Effects of Nature Therapy: A Review of Research in Japan," *International Journal of Environmental*

Research and Public Health 13, no. 8 (2016): E781, https://www.ncbi.nlm.nih.gov/pubmed/27527193/.

3 M. Igarashi, C. Song, H. Ikei, and Y. Miyazaki, "Effect of Stimulation by Foliage Plant Display Images on Prefrontal Cortex Activity: A Comparison with Stimulation Using Actual Foliage Plants," *Journal of Neuroimaging* 25, no. 1 (January–February 2015): 127–130.

CHAPTER 10: Reiki: Rituals for the Spirit

1 "The Legacy of Marcel Vogel," transcript of a paper presented at the 1996 Second Annual Advanced Water Sciences Symposium and the 1998 United States Psychotronics Association Conference, http://www.vogelcrystals.net/legacy_of_marcel_vogel.htm.

INDEX

natural materials, in your home, 134, 136
natural rhythm, finding your own, 58–
    60, 63
natural sleep hygiene, 123–25
nature, going outside into, 110, 120
    earth awakening and, 125–27
    earthing and, 128–30
    forest bathing *(shinrin-yoku)* and,
        258–59
    gardening and herbs and, 131–32
needs of others vs. ourselves, 145–46
negative energy, home detox ritual and,
    257–58
negative ions, 134
negative thoughts, 143–44, 146, 147, 174
new moon, ritual for, 263–65
nocebo effect, 148
not-doing, 60–63, 86–87

One Nation Under Stress, 7–8
outdoors, *see* nature, going outdoors into

pain, physical, iv, 104, 197, 214
    EFT and, 167, 168
    imprints surfacing as, 30–36
    Reiki and, 219, 220, 234–35
Palo Santo, 135
pendulum ritual, 261–63
personal hygiene, 153
pets:
    human bond with, 207
    Reiki for, 238–39
phone, checking as soon as you wake up,
    9, 152–53, 245
physical check-in, 110–11
physical exams, yearly, 108–9
physical intuition, 107–10
pictures, displayed in your home, 137
Pinker, Susan, 190, 192, 209
placebo effect, 148–49
positive thoughts:
    healing power of, 146–48
    mental hygiene and, 149–54
prana, 188, 212, 218, 219
prayer:
    before important event, 268
    power of, 210–11
Pure Barre, 33
purpose, 158–59

astrology and human design and,
    172–74
knowing your sense of, 93–94, 141,
    158–59, 176–80

quartz crystals, 278–79

Reiki, xiv, 33–35, 164, 168, 188, 197, 204,
    212, 218–24
    for anxiety, 235–36
    becoming a practitioner of, 226–27
    chakra balancing ritual, 272–76
    from a distance, 101, 210, 211, 240
    for exhaustion, 236–37
    for food, 221, 234, 237–38
    handwashing ritual, 269–70
    how to use, 233–34
    infusing space in home or hospital
        with, 234, 240
    learning to feel energy of, 230–33
    on loved one, 239–40
    for pain or injury, 234–35
    on pets, 238–39
    precepts of, 65–66, 223
    right before sleep, 236, 250
    ritual for feeling your energy, 270–72
    science of, 222
    starting your practice of, 224
    surrendering to yourself and, 44–47
    surrendering yourself to flow of
        energy in, 228–30
relationships, 198–206
    each person's imprints activated in,
        199
    ending, 206
    human-animal bond and, 207
    inner, with yourself, 202–3
    seeking control over other person in,
        199–200, 202
    setting boundaries in, 205
    thinking about, 181–82
    three types of, 201–2
    see also social connections
religious affiliation, 195, 196–97
repetitive thoughts, 143–44, 161
rhythm, natural, finding your own, 58–
    60, 63
rituals, 243–80
    afternoon tea ceremony, 248–49

ABOUT THE AUTHOR

KELSEY J. PATEL is a sought-after spiritual empowerment coach, Reiki healer, meditation and yoga teacher, EFT guide, and speaker. She teaches corporate workshops, leads retreats, holds one-on-one wellness sessions, and inspires and coaches audiences on manifesting their life goals nationally and internationally. Some of the hottest names and brands in Hollywood as well as leaders of Fortune 500 companies endorse her work.

Kelsey has dedicated her life to helping her clients live vibrant, joy-filled, abundant lives. Through her public speaking, consulting, workshops, classes, and private client sessions, she utilizes a range of techniques to help her clients recognize their own truths, release old patterns, and begin leading more authentic and fulfilling lives. Her students and clients say they have achieved more clarity, relaxation, purpose, awareness, inspiration, motivation, and healing from burnout.

Also the creator and owner of Magik Vibes, a spiritual and wellness product–based company that has been recognized by top media, Kelsey has owned various businesses, including a top-tier fitness studio and a clothing line, and has invested in other health- and wellness-related ventures. She teaches workshops at the DEN Meditation Center and Unplug in Los Angeles, and she was exclusively selected as the sole mindfulness ambassador for the lululemon flagship store in Beverly Hills. A hands-on and financial supporter of nonprofit organizations, including Dress for Success, Step Up Women's Network (LA Chapter board member), and No Kid Hungry, Kelsey is as committed to giving back as she is to changing lives. She lives in Los Angeles with her husband and two children.

To learn more, visit www.kelseyjpatel.com.